PCOS Repair Protocol

The complete manual to thriving with Polycystic Ovary Syndrome by uncovering the root cause of your symptoms

TAMIKA WOODS

Clinical Nutritionist and Fertility Educator

The information provided throughout this book is for educational purposes only. It is not a substitute for professional medical advice, diagnosis or treatment by a healthcare provider. Please consult with your healthcare practitioner before beginning any new supplement, exercise or lifestyle changes to make sure they are appropriate for you. If you have a medical problem or need medical advice, please see your doctor.

The names of some individuals have been changed to protect their identity.

First published in 2022 by Fire Publishing.

For further information visit the author's website at https://nourishednaturalhealth.com/

Instagram and Facebook: @Nourishednaturalhealth

For my darling daughter Sage.

You inspire me every day to make the world a better place for women.

Contents

Book Bonuses

To provide more depth and help you implement the advice covered in this book, I have created several free bonus resources for you which you will find mentioned throughout this book, as well as a free support community. You can access these resources at any time by heading to nourishednaturalhealth.com/resources

The bonus resources include:

PCOS Fertility Formula

Learn how to identify your fertile window and fall pregnant naturally with this four-part mini course.

Simple Weight Loss Strategies for PCOS

Scientifically proven strategies to lose weight sustainably and keep it off.

PCOS Supplement Protocol

Individualized supplement recommendations for your unique root cause.

Kick Your Sugar Cravings

The six-step formula to breaking up with sugar.

Beat the Bloat: 3 Hacks to Supercharged Digestion

Evidence-based solutions to support your digestive health.

PCOS-Friendly Food Formula

The complete manual to making any meal PCOS-friendly.

Acne & Hair Solutions Masterclass

Deep dive into the biggest secrets to reverse acne, unwanted hair growth, and hair thinning.

I need your help

If you find this book helpful it would mean so much to me if you leave a review on Amazon or Goodreads.

It is my life calling to get this information into the hands of as many women as physically (or digitally!) possible. I believe that all women deserve access to this life changing information.

By leaving a review you will help the women who need this book see that it can change their lives for the better. No matter what, I appreciate you and can't wait to continue to support you on your journey.

As you go through this book, don't forget to share your journey in our free PCOS Repair Cysterhood Community or tag me on Instagram @nourishednaturalhealth so that we can all cheer you on. Create your free Cysterhood Community account by navigating to nourishednaturalhealth.com/resources where you can join our thriving, supportive community of women rising above their PCOS diagnosis.

Foreword – Tam's PCOS Journey

Hey Cyster! Tamika Woods here – Clinical Nutritionist, Natural Fertility Educator, founder of Nourished Natural Health, and most importantly – a fellow Polycystic Ovary Syndrome (PCOS) Cyster. For those of you who are new to this term, the thriving community of women with PCOS often refer to each other as "Cysters".

My journey with PCOS started in my teens. Like many others, the acne around my jawline and irregular cycles prompted me to visit my doctor. Within minutes I was prescribed the pill as a "solution" to fix my period problems by regulating my period and clearing my skin. Fast forward four years of dealing with weekly migraines triggered by the pill, I decided to stop taking it and see how my body reacted.

To my surprise – all of my old symptoms came back! The migraines disappeared, but my period only showed up once every few months and my skin broke out worse than in my high school days. I was gaining weight just by *looking* at a piece of cake, I had zero energy and my anxiety levels skyrocketed. My gut flared up, and I was constantly bloated and feeling unwell.

I didn't want to leave the house because I was so embarrassed about my skin. I was constantly on edge not knowing when my period would arrive. My hair was falling out in clumps. I was ruining my relationship with my mood swings...

In short: I felt completely uncomfortable and ashamed to be in my own body.

So, I found myself back in the doctor's office, finally receiving a diagnosis of PCOS. I was told it would be very difficult to fall pregnant naturally in the future and that the best solution was to "lose some weight and exercise more." As a type-A overachiever, I took this information to the extreme.

I tried every fad diet out there. I did the juice cleanses. Intermittent fasting. Keto. Vegan. Low FODMAP. 5:2. Paleo.

I joined the gym and took the highest intensity classes they had on offer every morning. I hit the pavement in the evening and tried to "jog it off."

I bought every celebrity-endorsed face mask that promised to clear my skin. Spent thousands on vitamins that promised to regulate my cycle. Did clay cleanses to "detox" my gut.

But *nothing* was working.

My symptoms were getting worse. The weight wasn't budging. I was miserable, exhausted, and losing hope fast. I decided I needed to take matters into my own hands because the answers I needed weren't out there in my endless Google searches or influencer posts on Instagram.

I went back to university and spent nine years studying Nutritional Medicine, Education, and Women's Health and Fertility. During this time, it slowly dawned on me that the way I had been trying to address my PCOS was *completely wrong.*

I realized that I needed to address the *root cause* of my symptoms instead of treating each symptom separately. I had a burning desire to know *why* I was feeling the way I did.

I needed to understand what was holding me back from clearing my skin, regulating my cycle, finding a stable weight, and conceiving naturally in the future.

In my research, I discovered that there are four distinct types of PCOS that manifest in similar symptoms but are caused by different underlying root causes – unique to each woman.

Through testing and experimentation, I discovered that high stress hormones were at the heart of my personal PCOS symptoms. This meant that the high intensity workouts, following restrictive diets, and putting huge amounts of pressure on myself weren't just not helping my PCOS – they were actually making it *worse*!

It turns out the standard diet and exercise advice doesn't work for us PCOS Cysters. The way our bodies use glucose (sugar), burn calories, manage stress hormones, and control inflammation isn't the same as our non-PCOS friends. We need a specialized approach that supports our unique hormonal condition.

Over the next few years, I tested out protocols on myself and my one-to-one clients. I discovered that by addressing the root cause of PCOS as well as following specialized PCOS-friendly diet and lifestyle advice, it was possible to reverse the frustrating symptoms that come with this syndrome.

By 2019, I had cleared my skin, found a healthy, stable weight (without feeling deprived), was having regular, 29-day cycles, and *finally* felt like myself again. I had repaired my relationship, gotten married, and had a burning desire to share all of my knowledge with the world.

This is when my dream business Nourished Natural Health was born – a safe place for women to learn about the diet and lifestyle practices that support hormonal wellness. I developed the world-first PCOS Root Cause Vitamin Range to target the unique underlying causes of PCOS. You can check out the full range at shop.nourishednaturalhealth.com

In 2020, my husband and I fell pregnant naturally after only three months of trying, and I gave birth to my beautiful baby girl Sage in early 2021. After years of being told I would need drugs to fall pregnant, this felt like the ultimate testament to all my hard work.

After experiencing firsthand how the right targeted advice could completely resolve my symptoms and change my life, I knew I had to write this book and get this information into as many Cysters' hands as possible.

I took everything I had learned through my research, personal journey, and work with clients and developed the PCOS Repair Protocol: four simple, evidence-based steps to reverse your unique root cause. To date, this framework has already helped hundreds of women turn their lives around, reverse symptoms they thought they were stuck with, fall pregnant naturally, and thrive *with* PCOS, not in spite of it.

I've covered everything you need to know to create and implement your own individualized PCOS Repair Protocol within this book. I haven't left anything out. I want you to have access to this information so that you can transform your life.

Despite this, sometimes it can feel like you need help to piece the information together, work out where to start and actually stick to it. This is why I created the PCOS Repair Digital Program: an 8 week video course where I take you by the hand and guide you, step by step, through implementing the protocols in this book. The program is completely customized to your root cause which we identify in the first module. By individualizing the steps to follow within the program, you focus on only what is most impactful for your PCOS.

Members in the PCOS Repair Digital Program have access to my highly trained team of nutritionists and naturopaths to answer questions and make recommendations as you progress through the 8 weeks. As well as this, you receive tons of resources to support you on your journey including recipe books, workout videos, acne and hair guides, cycle tracking modules and fertility tips.

If you feel called to go deeper and received individualized support to help you make the changes in this book a reality, you can find out more about the program at nourishednaturalhealth.com/resources

Over the past few years, I have been fortunate enough to work with thousands of women with PCOS and other hormonal conditions to find the evidence-based advice that works for them to turn their lives around and start thriving again. I can't wait for you to be one of them.

Having PCOS is incredibly tough. It can feel unfair that we have all of these extra things to take care of when our friends seem to be able to live life however they please.

I like to remind myself that PCOS taught me the importance of self care. Without the acne, the hair loss, the weight changes, and the period problems, I would have never been inspired to take a deep look at the way I lived my life and took care of my body.

I am forever grateful for my PCOS in teaching me how to deeply listen and understand what my body needs, and respond with love. Being a Cyster has taught me incredible resilience and a deep compassion for other women.

It is my hope for you that, wherever you are on this journey, you can take solace in the fact that while PCOS is a lifelong condition, with the right advice, it is absolutely possible to live symptom-free. Having this condition has already made you stronger and more resilient and has brought you into one of the most supportive communities of women I have ever met.

There is a vibrant, balanced version of you deep inside (as much as it might not feel like it right now) and I cannot wait for you to meet her again.

Let's get started,
Tam.

Chapter 1

Welcome

For many of us, PCOS is tied to a feeling of restriction and deprivation after years spent trying to stick to diets and exercise plans in order to manage our symptoms. As you're reading this, an old familiar feeling of dread might be creeping in again. You might be wondering: "Will she tell me to cut out gluten, carbs, sugar, or dairy forever?" or "How much intense exercise will she tell me to do?".

When you were first diagnosed, you were likely told by your practitioner that to manage your PCOS, you need to "lose weight and exercise more." The problem with this statement is that, for women with PCOS who haven't addressed their root cause, *losing weight is almost impossible.* What's more, exercising harder can actually *worsen* PCOS symptoms.

Our bodies don't function the same as that of someone without PCOS. The reason that the diets and workout routines you've tried in the past haven't worked *isn't* because you failed to stick to the plan or you weren't disciplined enough.

Our hormonal imbalances prevent our bodies from shedding weight *even* when we eat less and move more. This is a protective measure because our body knows that our hormones are out of whack. Once we address what's causing your hormone imbalances and put a highly personalized plan in place, you will find that finding a healthy weight becomes a happy side effect of working on your root cause.

I have worked with hundreds of women who have felt like failures because they couldn't keep following ridiculously low calorie or restrictive diet plans. So many of these women told me they thought they were the problem.

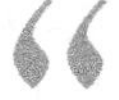

> If you've failed in the past, I want you to know:
> It isn't your fault.
> You're not a lost cause.
> Your body isn't broken.
> You're definitely not any less of a woman.
> And with the right advice, you *can* thrive with PCOS.

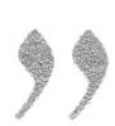

It *is* possible to easily achieve a healthy weight, clear your acne, regulate your cycles, stop excessive hair growth and fall pregnant naturally with PCOS.

You just need the right, individualized advice to reverse your root cause so that you can live your most incredible, symptom-free life.

The PCOS Repair Protocol does not involve deprivation diets, cutting out foods you love forever, killing yourself at the gym, or completely overhauling your lifestyle.

This is because those methods don't work.

On my own ten-year journey to find answers, I tried every diet under the sun and failed to lose weight, clear my skin, or get my periods regular again. Not only did I see no results, I was tired, cranky, snapping at my husband, and *literally consumed by thoughts about food* – it was exhausting!

I designed the PCOS Repair Protocol to focus on abundance rather than restriction. No foods are 100% off limits. You won't find a hardcore workout plan or lengthy daily practices you have to follow.

Over the next few chapters, you'll learn how you can focus on *increasing* the foods that are most supportive for your PCOS, so that you naturally crowd out less helpful foods without ever feeling deprived. You'll discover which specific changes will be most impactful for your unique PCOS root cause, and which you can get away with not following.

Together, we will create a plan that focuses on the minimal number of changes for maximum effect on your symptoms. The changes you make will be staggered so that you never feel overwhelmed with doing everything all at once.

We'll cover the top evidence-based hacks to transform your new routines into lifelong habits. Within a few months, not only will you be noticing a significant reduction in your symptoms, you will be effortlessly following the PCOS Repair Protocol principles and *finally* living in flow with your PCOS.

This journey will ultimately set you up for lifetime success. My team and I are here to support you in the long term, whether you choose to have our support through this book, through our free support community, or by working directly with us in our PCOS Repair Digital Program. Find out more at nourishednaturalhealth.com/resources

You'll find everything you need to heal the root cause of your PCOS in this book. I haven't held anything back because I want you to have the best chance to thrive with PCOS. Many Cysters have been able to completely turn their lives around simply by implementing the Protocol I outline in this book.

If you find you need more support in implementing these protocols and finding ways to help your new habits stick, my team and I are here for you.

It's time to take back control and thrive with PCOS!

Chapter 2

What is PCOS and How Did I Get It?

The name Polycystic Ovary Syndrome implies there is a problem with your ovaries, but really it's a *whole body disorder* that affects ovulation and causes your body to produce too many androgens (masculine hormones like testosterone). This causes symptoms like irregular or missing periods, acne, facial hair growth, thinning hair on your scalp, and weight gain.

There has been much debate about the name PCOS as it doesn't accurately describe what's going on in your body. For starters, the name was coined due to the "cyst-like appearance" of follicles seen on ultrasound scans. Researchers noticed women with PCOS often had ovaries that looked like a string of pearls – with lots of tiny, under-developed follicles. These "cysts" aren't really cysts at all, but multiple "baby eggs" that attempted to grow but never made it to full size.

It's common for baby eggs to begin developing but become stalled due to the hormonal imbalances associated with PCOS. Once the egg becomes stalled, your body decides to discard that baby egg and try again with a new one. It often takes several tries before your body is able to grow a full-sized egg and release this at ovulation. Once you have finally ovulated, this is followed by a period around two weeks later. This is why very long cycles or missing periods are a common feature of PCOS.

Interestingly, not all women with PCOS have polycystic ovaries. You can still meet the criteria for diagnosis based on other signs and symptoms including irregular cycles (more than 35 days between periods) and hyperandrogenism (high testosterone on blood tests and/or physical signs like acne and hirsutism).[1] In young women in particular, ultrasounds are an unreliable means of diagnosis as up to 70% of healthy women under 21 have polycystic ovaries.[2]

Since PCOS doesn't involve true cysts on your ovaries, and some women have normal ovaries on ultrasound, researchers have proposed several different names to more accurately describe what is going on in your body. Some of my personal favorites include "Metabolic Reproductive Syndrome" and "Metabolic Hyperandrogenic Syndrome."[3] For now, we'll stick to the name PCOS, but watch this space for updates!

PCOS is a *syndrome* not a singular disease. It is a group of symptoms related to too many androgens. Other syndromes you might have heard of include irritable bowel syndrome (IBS) and chronic fatigue syndrome (CFS). What's common between these syndromes is that they describe a group of symptoms, which can have multiple root causes.

Let's think about an IBS scenario for a minute. Sarah developed IBS because she caught a stomach bug whilst on holiday in Thailand and ended up with a parasite infection. Tara has IBS because she works a highly stressful job and drinks lots of coffee on an empty stomach to keep up with the workload.

Both Sarah and Tara experience painful bloating, alternating diarrhea and constipation, and stomach cramps. However, the treatment that will help resolve their symptoms is likely completely different. Sarah might benefit from a course of antibiotics to kill the parasite, while Tara might benefit from learning stress management techniques and swapping coffee for green tea.

Syndromes don't have one simple test that can be used to diagnose them. Similarly, syndromes don't have one singular medication or procedure that will work for everyone because the root cause is different in each case. If you have been officially diagnosed with PCOS, this is because you met a specific criteria of symptoms. To understand what is *causing* these symptoms, we need to look deeper.

You might be experiencing your PCOS symptoms because of your body's sensitivity to stress hormones. It could be a combination of your genetics making your insulin function less efficiently as well as eating a diet that doesn't support your blood sugar levels. You might have increased levels of inflammation in your body due to an underlying food sensitivity that has gone unaddressed. Or you might have recently stopped taking the birth control pill, causing a temporary overproduction of androgens in your ovaries.

This is why a very low carb or ketogenic diet worked for a PCOS influencer you saw on Instagram, but you felt worse when you tried it. Or why your friend with PCOS feels amazing after an early morning

HIIT class, but your energy is tanked for the rest of the day. In the same way that we need to know *why* someone is experiencing IBS in order to prescribe the right treatment, to truly heal your PCOS, we first need to understand your root cause.

In my many years working with women with PCOS, I discovered that there are four distinct root causes (or "types") of PCOS:

1. Insulin resistance
2. Adrenal (stress-based)
3. Inflammatory
4. Post-birth control.

For a Cyster with insulin-resistant PCOS and no issues with her adrenal glands or stress hormones, a very low carb diet and high intensity exercise plan could be incredibly helpful in reversing her symptoms. For another Cyster with adrenal PCOS, the same plan could leave her feeling moody, stressed, hungry, and with no improvement in her symptoms.

Over the next few chapters, you'll discover exactly which one (or combination) of these four root causes is driving your symptoms. We will then create an individualized, step-by-step plan to reverse your PCOS type. We'll identify the most important food, movement, mindset, and supplement changes to address your unique root cause and reverse your symptoms for good, so you can start thriving with PCOS.

How did I get PCOS?

Research in this area is still developing, however at this point in time, there seem to be three key influences that increase your risk of developing PCOS: genetics, endocrine development, and environmental exposure. When researchers examined families of women with PCOS, they found that both male and female relatives were much more likely to have metabolic syndrome, insulin resistance, high blood pressure, and high cholesterol.[4] This suggests that there may be a familial genetic link involved with the development of PCOS.

Research has also shown that early exposure to endocrine disrupting chemicals like pesticides, phthalates and Bisphenol A (BPA) as a fetus or in early childhood may impact the development of your hypothalamus-pituitary-ovarian axis (the way your brain talks to your ovaries).[5] This can lead to issues with ovulation and increased production of androgens, causing the symptoms of PCOS. Increased stress hormones and chronic dieting in the years before and during puberty have also been linked with an increased risk of developing PCOS later in life.[6]

Finally, there are several environmental triggers that have been shown to accelerate or "switch on" your development of PCOS. These include insulin resistance, inflammation, and stress hormones.[7] In some women, taking the oral contraceptive pill can also temporarily trigger the symptoms of PCOS due to a surge in androgens.

Think about it like this: You are born with an increased likelihood of developing PCOS, and then certain triggers in your environment and your lifestyle cause that gene to be switched on, leading to the symptoms of PCOS. While we can't change your genetics or what happened in your early life, we *can* change your current environment to minimize the expression of your PCOS and eventually reverse your symptoms.

How does my root cause create my PCOS symptoms?

Women with PCOS have an increased likelihood of making too many androgens and having problems with ovulation due to their family history. Over time, certain things in life "switch on" our PCOS gene.

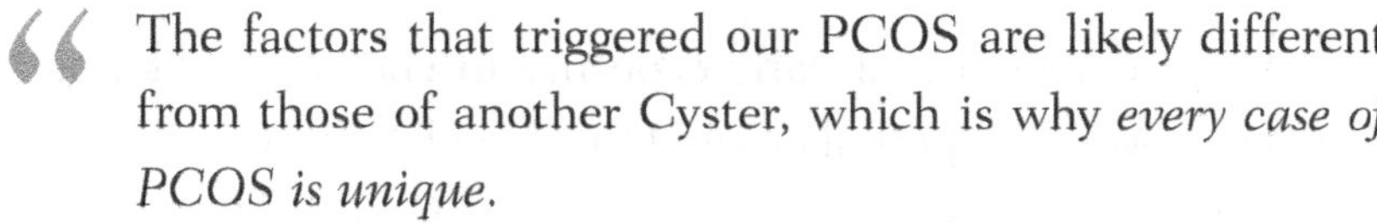

> "The factors that triggered our PCOS are likely different from those of another Cyster, which is why *every case of PCOS is unique.*"

At the heart of it, your unique root cause stimulates your body to produce too much testosterone or other androgens. The way this happens depends on which root cause of PCOS (or combination) you are dealing with.

High levels of insulin or having inflammation for a long time causes your ovaries to produce too much testosterone. High levels of stress hormones cause your adrenal glands to produce more adrenal androgens. Imbalances in your thyroid hormones trigger increased testosterone production and can impact ovulation.

Testosterone gets into the oil glands under your skin, particularly around your chin and jawline, and causes excess sebum (skin oil) production. This extra oil blocks your hair follicles and causes an infection, leading to those frustrating spots we know as pimples.

In some women, the fine, soft hairs known as vellus hairs on your chin, upper lip, breasts, lower abdomen, inner thighs, and lower back are hormone sensitive. This means that when you have high levels of testosterone, these hairs change from vellus hairs to terminal hairs – long, coarse and dark hairs which grow much faster (and mean you need to shave or wax *constantly*). This situation is known as hirsutism and commonly includes the thinning of hair on your scalp.

Scalp hair follies are also hormone sensitive, but instead of becoming terminal hairs, testosterone is converted into dihydrotestosterone (DHT) – a very potent version of testosterone. DHT causes the hair follicles to die and fall out – leading to thinning hair on your head.

As well as causing acne and hair changes, insulin, testosterone, stress hormones, chronic inflammation, and thyroid imbalances can all disrupt your ovulation and periods. This can lead to very long cycles or missing periods altogether.

If you aren't having regular periods, your doctor might have talked to you about the importance of bleeding regularly and may have prescribed medication like the pill or the Depo Provera shot to artificially induce a bleed. This is because going for long periods of time without shedding your endometrial lining (which is what happens when you bleed on your period), may increase your risk of endometrial cancer.

While regular bleeds are important, regular ovulation is arguably even more critical because this is how we keep our heart, bones, and breast tissue healthy. Not ovulating can significantly impact your bone density as well as increase your risk of cardiovascular disease.[8]

By addressing your root cause, you can support your body to start ovulating naturally and having regular cycles again. Not only will this improve your lifelong disease risk, but it will also mean that you are having regular, natural bleeds without the need for medication. This is because ovulation is always followed by a period bleed (unless you're pregnant).

Can the pill regulate my cycle or fix my symptoms?

There is a common misconception that the birth control pill can "regulate your cycle." This is because, when you follow the pill schedule on the packet, your period magically arrives every 28 days, creating a false sense of regularity. In reality, the bleed you have whilst on the pill is caused by a withdrawal from the synthetic hormones, rather than due to ovulation.

A normal cycle involves ovulation, followed by (if you're not pregnant) the shedding of the lining of your uterus in the form of your period roughly two weeks later. In contrast, the pill works by shutting down ovulation in order to prevent pregnancy.

In the final week of most pill packets, you will find placebo tablets. They are often marked by a different color. These tablets are "inactive" – meaning they don't contain synthetic hormones. There is actually no need to consume these tablets, however manufacturers add them to the packet to help you keep the routine of swallowing a pill each day.

The reason these placebo tablets are there is to cause a temporary withdrawal from the synthetic hormones that trigger your endometrial lining to shed. This is the bleed that looks like a period.

Whilst it can feel like the pill has fixed your irregular cycles because you are bleeding regularly, the reality is that you still have not addressed the root cause of why you aren't ovulating. This means that when you stop taking the pill, your irregular cycles will very likely return.

Hormonal birth control can also be very helpful in managing some of the other frustrating symptoms of PCOS like acne and hair changes. These symptoms are caused by high levels of testosterone and other androgens. Certain brands of the pill have strong anti-androgenic effects – meaning they block the effects of high testosterone. This is why you may have been offered the pill as a "solution" to your symptoms by your doctor.

Unfortunately, while the pill can block the effects of testosterone temporarily, it cannot teach your body to produce less. This means that once you stop taking the pill, these symptoms will likely reappear and often more severely than before.

While the pill and other medications absolutely have a place in supporting severe symptoms, I want you to choose these medications informed with the knowledge that they are temporary, band-aid solutions. I know all too well that sometimes we just need a break from the debilitating symptoms of PCOS.

I have used the pill and other medications myself out of desperation, and I am grateful that they were there when I needed them. However, when you are ready to reverse your symptoms for good, it's time to *address your root cause.*

This isn't going to be an overnight fix, but putting some targeted strategies in place now to support your unique PCOS type will greatly improve your symptoms, boost your fertility, and reduce your lifelong disease risk. Plus, you'll likely experience other bonus "side effects" like increased energy, smooth digestion, improved moods, better sleep, and increased libido!

The principles you will learn in this book will support your body for the rest of your life, not just for a few weeks or months. I cannot wait for you to experience how empowering it is to finally understand what your body needs and create a lifestyle that supports this.

What will happen if I don't address my root cause?

If you don't address *why* your body is producing too many androgens and having issues with ovulation, your symptoms probably won't improve and will likely get worse over time. You may also increase your risk of developing more severe conditions over time.

Let's look at some issues that can happen with each root cause if it goes unaddressed for a long time. I've provided these points to keep you informed and to motivate you – not to scare you. It's important to understand what putting the work in now can mean for your future.

Just because these risks are listed for your root cause does not mean you are destined to experience them. If you take action now to take charge of your PCOS, you can dramatically reduce your risk of the conditions mentioned below.

Insulin resistance

Research indicates that around 70% of people with insulin resistance go on to develop type 2 diabetes when left untreated. Type 2 diabetes significantly impacts your entire body – from eyesight to blood vessels, blood flow to your feet, sexual function, heart, nerves, and kidneys. It also increases your risk of developing heart disease and certain cancers.

Having high insulin also heightens your risk of pregnancy complications if your insulin is not under control during pregnancy. Studies show a 24% increased risk of preeclampsia and around a 40% increased risk of gestational diabetes for women with high insulin.[9] High insulin has been shown to reduce the effectiveness of certain fertility drugs like letrozole and clomid.[10]

If conceiving in the future is a priority for you, improving your insulin resistance now will have dramatic effects on both your ability to conceive and to have a healthy pregnancy with fewer complications.

Less life threatening, but still hugely impactful on your quality of life, suffering from insulin resistance causes rollercoaster fluctuations in energy, sugar and carbohydrate cravings as well as brain fog, "hangry' attacks," mood swings and stubborn weight gain (particularly around your midsection). Having experienced imbalanced blood sugar levels myself, I cannot overstate the night and day difference of getting this under control.

Before I addressed my insulin resistance, I couldn't go two hours without a meal or snack. If I did, I would end up shaking, lightheaded, cranky, and not able to think straight. This meant I had to constantly think ahead, pack my snacks, and know where and when I would be eating next.

I also dealt with overwhelming sugar cravings after every meal and felt like I was *always* thinking about food. My thoughts were consumed by food, and I found myself thinking of what sweet treat I would eat before I even finished my main meals.

Healing your insulin resistance now will dramatically improve your lifelong disease risk, significantly lower your risk of pregnancy complications, support you to find a healthy weight, *and* stop cravings from ruling your headspace and energy levels.

High stress hormones

Back in caveman times, cortisol and adrenaline were the hormones our body used in short bursts to give us energy to escape danger. Our adrenal glands dump glucose into our bloodstream to help power our muscles to run away or fight a predator.

This system works really well when you are dealing with occasional threats to your survival that require you to run fast. The problem with modern-day stress is that we very rarely experience stress from a physical threat.

More often, our stress is experienced sitting at a desk with a demanding boss or running late and stuck in the car in traffic. Rather than in a short burst, we often experience stress relentlessly.

This means that, over time, our body continues dumping glucose into our bloodstream to help us run or fight, but we aren't using the energy. This extra glucose can cause our bodies to become less responsive to insulin, eventually leading to insulin resistance.

Chronically high cortisol impairs your immune system function, making it harder to fight off infections and increasing your recovery time. This is because our bodies are prioritizing keeping us safe from the immediate stress, rather than fighting viruses or infections.

Running off adrenaline can feel really good at the time and can actually be quite addictive. There have been many periods of my life where I have run off a couple of hours of broken sleep, way too much coffee, and the buzz of looming deadlines.

For a while you can feel superhuman and tick so many things off your to-do list. However, over time, our adrenal glands can't keep up with the constant output of cortisol and we end up feeling "tired but wired."

This is where your energy levels go from sky-high to rock bottom for the majority of the day. All of a sudden, you may struggle to complete normal tasks or even get out of bed without caffeine. You never feel refreshed, even after a full night's sleep, and struggle to deal with normal levels of exercise or stress.

You find yourself wandering around during the day in a foggy haze, then, often right before bedtime, you experience a sudden surge of energy that can prevent you from sleeping, further worsening your fatigue.

I've personally experienced complete burnout in my energy levels after asking too much of my adrenals and had to take significant steps to recover. You can reverse this situation, however it is significantly more difficult once you are already depleted. If we can address your stress hormones *before* you get to rock bottom, it will be a much simpler and faster process.

Inflammation

Chronically high levels of inflammation increases your risk of developing certain autoimmune conditions like rheumatoid arthritis, Hashimoto's thyroiditis, and Lupus.[11] It also increases the likelihood of experiencing inflammatory conditions like hypertension, poor mental health, and cardiovascular disease.

Not all inflammation is "bad." Inflammation is a necessary part of our immune system and we want it in small amounts to help our body fight acute infections and deal with injuries. Our body uses inflammation to send immune cells to parts of the body that need help fighting foreign invaders (like a virus) and to heal damaged tissue.

In a healthy inflammatory situation, an event triggers increased inflammation – for example, contracting the common cold. The immune system mounts its response, kills the virus, and we get better. Now that the threat has passed, we can switch off the inflammation and go back to normal.

The problem with our modern lifestyle is that the inflammation doesn't switch off after the threat disappears. This means our immune system doesn't have a chance to rest and recover before the next event. When it is chronically activated, our immune system can become tired and confused and start to attack our own tissues instead of just foreign invaders. This is what leads to autoimmune diseases like those mentioned earlier.

By addressing the cause of your increased inflammation now (for example, poor gut health, food intolerances, or low vitamin and mineral levels), you can dramatically reduce the chances of your immune system becoming overstimulated and developing the conditions above.

ACTION STEP:

Share your biggest takeaways from this chapter in the PCOS Repair Cysterhood Community. If you haven't joined our community, head to nourishednaturalhealth.com/resources to sign up for free.

Chapter 3

The Four-Step PCOS Repair Protocol to Reverse the Root Cause of Your PCOS

The four-step framework I am about to share with you was born out of years of working with Cysters to heal the root cause of their PCOS. This exact framework has helped thousands of women stop living life controlled by their symptoms, clear cystic acne, lose weight easily (and keep it off), reverse hair loss, and fall pregnant naturally.

This is in complete contrast to how I see most women start their PCOS journey (including myself). Time and time again, I see Cysters falling down the same traps in a desperate attempt to fix their symptoms. I call it the "Symptomatic Treatment Spiral." It goes a little like this: You know something is up because your skin is breaking out like a teenager, your period has gone MIA, and there is hair growing in places it *definitely* shouldn't be. So, you go to see your doctor.

The doctor diagnoses you with PCOS and tells you your only option is to lose weight, exercise more, take the pill, and come back for fertility treatment when you are ready to get pregnant. You leave the doctor's office feeling disheartened and scared about your future. You decide you'll do everything you can to get your health back on track.

So, you scour the internet for the latest diet hack or workout plan that seems to be working for other women. You start a new restrictive diet and exercise plan, cut out all the foods you love, and feel deprived, hungry, and exhausted.

You likely last a few days on the new plan, feel miserable, and see zero changes in your symptoms. You wonder why it seems so easy for everyone else. And so, you find yourself back on social media searching for the next potential "cure." This spiral continues for months or even years before you find yourself back in the doctor's office, feeling worse than before and being offered another medication to manage your symptoms.

At this point, it's common to feel like a failure. To wonder why you can't figure all of this out. To feel like your body is "broken" and fighting against you. The symptomatic treatment spiral not only sucked but also kept me stuck for more than ten years – forcing me to spend all my savings and time on finding a solution.

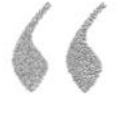

Here's how the PCOS Repair Protocol is different: Every single step is individualized to *your* unique root cause.

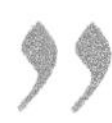

You won't find any one-size-fits-all solutions or claims that aren't backed by science. The Protocol doesn't involve dieting, calorie counting, exhausting workout plans, or completing overhauling your lifestyle. This is because these traditional methods *don't work* for women with PCOS.

We know from the research that women with PCOS have a different hormonal makeup and need specialized protocols to support this.

The PCOS Repair Protocol is informed by hundreds of research studies on the most impactful diet and lifestyle changes for PCOS, combined with the results I've gathered while working with my one-to-one clients for years. This book will give you the exact tools you need to identify and reverse your root cause for good, without ever feeling deprived or overwhelmed.

Here's the exact four-step protocol you'll be implementing over the next few chapters:

Step One – Quickly relieve symptoms by reducing androgens

PCOS causes our bodies to make too many androgens ("masculine" hormones like testosterone). This is the cause of the frustrating symptoms like acne, irregular cycles, hair loss on your head, and unwanted hair growth. In this first step, you'll learn how to quickly reduce your body's overproduction of androgens to give you relief from your symptoms while we dig deeper and heal your root cause. You'll notice clearer skin, more energy in the mornings, improved digestion, and fewer sugar cravings and hangry attacks.

Step Two – Uncover the Root Cause of Your PCOS

We'll deep dive into the four most common root causes of PCOS and work out which one (or combination) is driving your symptoms. This eye-opening step is often the "lightbulb" moment for Cysters because they finally see what has been holding them back from truly healing.

Step Three – Treat the Root Cause of Your PCOS

Now that you know what's driving your PCOS, it's time to implement an individualized protocol to address your unique root cause. This is the core of your treatment and the chunkiest step. I'll guide you every step of the way through which changes will be most impactful for you to make. Once you have reversed your root cause, your body will stop over-producing androgens.

Step Four – Find a Community and Thrive with PCOS

PCOS is a lifelong condition. This means the principles you'll learn in steps one to three will become habits you'll follow for the rest of your life, not just a few weeks or months. Having a community to lift you up when times are tough, cheer you on when you have breakthroughs, and inspire you to keep going is crucial. I'll provide you with a community of women to connect with as part of this book and explain how you can gain direct access to our team to support you at every step.

STEP ONE: Block Androgens for Quick Symptom Relief

PCOS causes our bodies to produce too many androgens ("male" hormones like testosterone). These cause frustrating and embarrassing symptoms like acne, hair thinning, excess hair growth, irregular cycles, and weight gain.

While ultimately we want to identify what is triggering your body to over-produce androgens (your "PCOS Root Cause") and reverse it, this takes time. In the short term, blocking the effects of excess androgens can help with symptom relief.

I like to think of this as similar to having a bad headache every day. You want to work out what's causing your headache, but the pain is so severe that you can't think straight. First, you might take some paracetamol to temporarily block the pain of the headache. Then, while you are experiencing relief from your symptoms, you can focus on what's causing your headache (for example – drinking too much coffee, your neck being out of alignment, or being too stressed).

Having this clarity allows you to work out the root cause of the headache, and then take steps to improve your symptoms. Ultimately, you won't get headaches anymore because you have solved *why* you were getting them. Paracetamol has gone from being a daily essential to something that sits on the shelf for only when you *really* need it.

Ta-da! You have treated the root cause of your headaches for lasting symptom relief.

I added this step into the PCOS Repair Protocol because after experiencing the humiliating symptoms of PCOS for more than a decade, I know how difficult it is to go about your day-to-day life and not just focus on your symptoms. I've spent long periods of my life feeling too embarrassed to leave the house because my skin was breaking out, my energy levels were tanked, and I felt so bloated and unwell.

By getting some quick wins with your symptoms, I know you will be motivated to dig deeper and work on your root cause. You won't need to follow these anti-androgen principles forever – they will just be helpful in the short term until you have found a lifestyle plan that works for you and your root cause. Once you are confidently implementing your individualized protocol, your body will stop over-producing androgens and you will likely no longer need the principles in this chapter.

The PCOS Repair Protocol approach requires you to think about what is actually going on with your body and question *why* you are getting symptoms. It will require more effort in the short term, but ultimately, it will serve as a solution for the rest of your life.

Chapter 4

The Anti-Androgen Plan

The first step in the PCOS Repair Protocol is to block the effects of excess androgens in your body so that you can find some relief from symptoms while we dig deeper into your root cause. You'll follow three simple daily rituals to improve your symptoms while we work on your root cause.

How do you know if you have excess androgens?

It's common for your doctor to run a blood test to check your testosterone levels when you have PCOS. If you've had this test recently, it may have come back with a higher than normal result. If this is the case, you can confidently assume excess testosterone is a key factor triggering your PCOS symptoms.

But what if your blood testosterone results are normal or on the lower side?

Many women that I work with have received normal or even low testosterone results in their blood work, yet suffer from significant androgen excess symptoms. There are a few reasons for this.

Firstly, testosterone is difficult to measure in your blood. A blood test for testosterone is only able to measure the testosterone that is circulating around your body. This doesn't let us see how much testosterone is bound up in your tissues – for example, trapped in your hair follicles causing acne, excess hair growth, or thinning of the hair on your head.

Secondly, testosterone is just one of the many androgens that cause the symptoms of PCOS. Testosterone is the most common androgen, which is why it is most frequently measured by your doctor. In your unique type of PCOS, your symptoms may be driven by another kind of androgen (like DHEAS, which is commonly raised when you experience high levels of stress).

Lastly, a testosterone blood test doesn't take into account how strongly an enzyme called 5-alpha reductase is working in your body. This enzyme is responsible for turning testosterone into a similar but much more potent form called dihydrotestosterone (DHT). Like testosterone, DHT gets into the hair follicles and causes acne, hirsutism, and hair thinning.[12]

The 5-alpha reductase enzyme has been shown to be around four times more active in women with PCOS than controls.[12] This means that even with normal levels of testosterone, your body may be far more efficient at converting testosterone to DHT, contributing to symptoms of PCOS.

The best way to assess for high androgen levels is to look at your symptoms. This is a much more reliable way of confirming if androgens are an issue in your PCOS symptoms. The most common symptoms to look out for are:

- Acne around your chin, jawline, upper lip, neck, chest, and back
- Thinning hair in the crown of your head or a widening part
- Receding hairline
- Extensive hair growth around your chin, neck, jawline, chest, breasts or back.

The Three Step Anti-Androgen Plan

Each day, follow these three simple rituals to reduce your symptoms, increase your energy, and reduce sugar cravings:

1. Drink two cups of spearmint tea.
2. Enjoy a PCOS Repair Breakfast.
3. Take an anti-androgen supplement.

Daily Ritual One: Drink Two Cups of Spearmint Tea

Spearmint tea has been shown to naturally lower androgens levels in women with PCOS.[13] In a randomized controlled trial, drinking two cups daily for 30 days resulted in lowered blood testosterone levels, improved LH to FSH ratios, and significantly reduced abnormal hair growth (hirsutism).[14] At this point in time, peppermint tea has not been studied so for best results seek out a spearmint tea (loose leaf or tea bags are both great choices).

Your goal is to enjoy two cups of spearmint tea daily to support balanced androgen levels. Get creative with this! You don't just have to drink hot tea. Try making a big batch and cooling in the fridge. Use cooled tea as a base for smoothies instead of milk, or freeze into cubes and add to water for a refreshing, cool drink.

Daily Ritual Two: Follow The PCOS Repair Breakfast Principles

Your second daily ritual is to enjoy a PCOS-friendly breakfast. We'll cover exactly what this means and how to tweak your existing breakfast to fit these principles in the next chapter.

Daily Ritual Three: Take an Androgen Blocking Supplement

Your final daily ritual is to take an androgen blocking supplement. This step is optional as the first two steps will go a long way in providing relief from some of your symptoms. However, for faster results, I suggest considering one of the following options. I recommend discussing any new supplement regimes with your primary care physician before beginning to be sure it is the best choice for you.

There are many herbs and vitamins that naturally help your body to balance androgen levels and reduce the conversion of testosterone to DHT, therefore improving your PCOS symptoms. Some of my favorite choices include those listed below.

Natural androgen blocking nutrients:

- **Saw palmetto →** reduces 5-alpha reductase activity and promotes estrogen balance

- **Reishi mushroom →** blocks DHT conversion in the hair and skin follicles, reducing excessive hair growth
- **Stinging nettle leaf →** increases sex hormone binding globulin (SHBG), which mops up excess androgens in the blood[15]
- **Zinc →** reduces acne formation and helps wound healing of existing acne scars
- **Shiitake mushroom →** improves insulin resistance, the root cause of at least 80% of PCOS cases
- **Maitake mushroom →** stimulates ovulation in women with PCOS who have irregular cycles almost as strongly as Clomiphene (the leading ovulation drug used in fertility clinics).[16]

I have used a combination of the supplements listed above for many years with my clients and seen dramatic improvements to stubborn acne, frustrating hair growth, thinning hair, and irregular ovulation.

While their results were incredible, my clients got sick of taking handfuls of pills each day, so I created *Nourished Androgen Blocker* – a single capsule containing the ideal ratio of natural androgen blocking nutrients in a convenient once a day dose.

Nourished Androgen Blocker was created based on research studies showing these ingredients powerfully lower high androgen levels,[17] slow testosterone conversion to DHT,[18] improve acne,[19] and promote regular ovulation.

You can find out more about Nourished Androgen Blocker at nourishednaturalhealth.com/resources

Please note that as Androgen Blocker contains herbal ingredients, it is not recommended during pregnancy or breastfeeding. Luckily, we have another alternative for Cysters who are currently on a fertility journey - Cycle Regulate + Ovulate. An Inositol supplement can be taken alongside Androgen Blocker or on its own.

Inositol is a nutrient similar in structure to a B-vitamin that has been studied extensively for its ability to improve irregular cycles, increase insulin sensitivity, promote ovulation, and enhance egg quality.[20] It has also been shown to regulate androgen levels, supporting a reduction of acne and hirsutism. If you struggle with irregular cycles, are planning to conceive in the near future, or are currently pregnant or breastfeeding, you will benefit from adding inositol to your regime, no matter which PCOS type you have.

I recommend Nourished Cycle Regulate + Ovulate because it contains the ideal 40:1 ratio of two forms of inositol: myo-inositol and D-chiro inositol – a similar ratio to what is found in the human body. A 2017 study that compared this 40:1 inositol combination with Metformin found the inositol group had significantly more weight loss, resumption of ovulation, and natural pregnancy than the Metformin group.[21] Inositol has very few side effects and is considered safe to consume whilst trying to conceive, during pregnancy, and whilst breastfeeding. It is also considered safe to take alongside Metformin as it works in a different way to improve your body's sensitivity to insulin. However, please always run any new supplement by your doctor for individualized advice before beginning.

You can find out more and purchase Cycle Regulate + Ovulate via nourishednaturalhealth.com/resources

ACTION STEP:

Share how you are drinking your spearmint tea in our PCOS Repair Cysterhood Community (and check out other Cysters' creative ideas!) If you haven't joined our community, head to nourishednaturalhealth.com/resources to sign up for free.

Chapter 5

The PCOS Repair Breakfast Principles

What you eat for breakfast is *the most impactful habit you can change for your PCOS*. More than any other meal of the day, your breakfast can either dramatically improve or worsen your symptoms. Simple tweaks can significantly reduce cravings and improve your energy levels, mood, and focus for the rest of your day. It can also boost your metabolism, support your body to find a healthy weight without feeling deprived, promote regular ovulation, and help lower the production of androgens.

Let's take a look at some of the most common breakfast meals: cereal, toast, fruit, and oatmeal. What these meals all have in common is that they are high in carbohydrates and low in protein. The carbohydrates in these foods are broken down into glucose (sugar) in your blood. This glucose needs to be stored in your cells for when you need energy later.

The hormone insulin is responsible for mopping up all of the sugar in your blood and telling your cells to open their doors and let the glucose in to be stored. I like to think of insulin as your taxi driver and the cell as your home. The insulin taxi picks you (the glucose) up and drives you home. Once you get home, your very courteous taxi driver gets out and knocks on your front door to let you inside.

In a normal situation, the door opens straight away and lets you inside. You can go inside, rest, and come back out when you are needed next. For women with PCOS, it's common for the taxi driver to knock and knock without any answer.

Because the door isn't opening, your taxi driver gets on the phone to some of their other taxi driver friends and asks them to come over and help. The other taxi drivers arrive and together they all knock on the door louder than before. Finally, the door swings open and you are able to go inside.

This analogy describes what's called *insulin resistance*. This is estimated to affect at least 80% of women with PCOS, contributing to many of its hallmark symptoms like weight gain, acne, and irregular cycles. Because our cells have become a little deaf to the door knocks from insulin, our bodies send out more and more insulin to have the same effect on our blood sugar levels. Having high insulin levels triggers your ovaries to produce more testosterone, worsening the symptoms of PCOS and making it harder for you to lose weight.

When this has gone on for a while, it's common for your body to send out far too much insulin all at once when you eat a higher carbohydrate meal. Insulin is really efficient at mopping up all the glucose in your blood, causing your blood sugar levels to drop quickly.

This sudden drop in blood sugar might cause you to feel jittery, hungry, moody, or low in energy soon after eating a standard breakfast like cereal or toast. This drop in blood sugar is called reactive hypoglycemia and it is very common for women with PCOS.

Eating a higher carbohydrate, lower protein breakfast places our blood sugar on a rollercoaster for the rest of the day. You might notice you are starving or really low in energy within a couple of hours of breakfast and find yourself snacking on sugar or caffeine to get you through the rest of the day.

Before I adopted the PCOS Repair Breakfast, I ate what I thought was a "super healthy" breakfast every morning for years. It was a smoothie made with lots of frozen banana, oats, and yogurt. Even though I felt really full after drinking this, within an hour or two, I would be *STARVING*. Like "get me to the nearest cafe before I do something crazy" kind of starving.

I'd spend the rest of the day snacking on sugary treats or crackers and drinking coffee to survive my plummeting energy levels. I felt grumpy, moody, and shaky if I didn't eat every two hours and was constantly preoccupied with when and where I'd be getting my next meal.

When I switched to the PCOS Repair Breakfast, I found that not only was I satisfied until lunchtime, I also had no more cravings for sugar for the *entire* rest of the day – even after dinner! I couldn't believe how switching up one meal could so significantly impact the rest of my day. These principles have been a game changer for so many of my clients over the years who have been able to achieve massive results just through this one simple change.

Even if you don't experience the symptoms of insulin resistance like increased hunger (if you've ever felt "hangry," you know what I mean!), weight gain around your middle, rollercoaster energy, or sugar or carb cravings, you will still benefit from following the PCOS Repair Breakfast principles. The PCOS Repair Breakfast is helpful even if you are underweight or don't have any issues with insulin resistance.

This is because eating a higher carbohydrate meal like toast, cereal, fruit, or oatmeal causes your body to produce more insulin to bring your blood sugar levels back down. Insulin causes our ovaries to produce more androgens, worsening your PCOS symptoms. Following the PCOS Repair Breakfast principles will help to balance your hormone levels, no matter which root cause of PCOS you are dealing with.

Unlike a higher carbohydrate meal, enjoying a high protein breakfast first thing in the morning is one of the best ways to keep your blood sugar levels stable. Protein-rich foods don't cause a large spike in your blood sugar levels, which means your body doesn't need to release as much insulin.

Eating this way assists the effects of your overnight fast without skipping breakfast (more on why that's not a good idea in the FAQs below). Protein is also extremely satiating, meaning it keeps you feeling full and satisfied for a long time.

When you follow these principles, you should feel full for at least three to four hours (and sometimes even up to six or seven hours). If you find you are feeling hungry after two hours, you might benefit from adding more healthy fats to your breakfast (like avocado, nut butter, or coconut milk).

The PCOS Repair Breakfast is essentially a high protein, low starch, and low sugar breakfast. You are going to be aiming for 30-40 grams of protein, along with lots of non-starchy vegetables and some healthy fat.

This means no starchy vegetables (like potato, sweet potato, or pumpkin), no grains (like oats, bread, cereal, or rice), and no legumes (like chickpeas or baked beans). You can enjoy a serve of berries as well as the other low sugar fruits listed below as these are naturally low in sugar and high in fiber, but avoid other fruits not listed at breakfast time. The exception to the no legume principle is tofu as this is naturally low in starch and high in protein. As a vegetarian option, tofu can be a great option to help you hit the 30-40g protein target. Always look for organic, non-GMO tofu to avoid potentially endocrine-disrupting chemicals in the sprays used on soy crops.

Don't worry – you are *not* cutting these foods out of your diet, and you will be able to include them in other meals during the day. After years of trialing different diet tweaks with my PCOS clients and myself, I have found that avoiding these foods in your first meal of the day is incredibly impactful.

For now, I just want you to focus on changing your breakfast. Don't worry about any of your other meals or snacks – we'll cover those a little later. This way of eating is likely going to feel very new to you, especially if you are used to eating a "standard" breakfast, or maybe not eating any breakfast at all. I want you to go easy on yourself as you start to follow these principles.

If you are struggling to meet the protein target, I suggest starting with a smaller amount of protein (like 20 grams) and slowly working your way up from there. After eating this way for a few weeks, you will notice that your hunger, fullness, and taste buds start to adapt.

One of the easiest ways to get your 30-40 grams of protein is to use a high quality protein powder. See the FAQs below for my top tips on choosing a PCOS-friendly protein powder if you would like to use one. Other great breakfast sources of protein include eggs, salmon, bacon, sausage or even leftover meats from the night before!

My biggest tip to help you implement these PCOS Repair Breakfast principles is to focus on vegetables that grow above the ground. These vegetables tend to be much lower in starch, and therefore they don't impact our blood sugar levels. They are also great swaps for some of the traditional carbs you are used to eating.

For example, frozen cauliflower or zucchini are great swaps for fruit in a smoothie. Try blending your favorite flavored protein powder (like vanilla or chocolate) with some frozen cauliflower or zucchini, plus some almond or coconut milk. Or replace the toast you usually have with your eggs with some sauteed greens like kale or spinach.

If you are finding the protein volume overwhelming, try mixing up your protein sources so that you are not having a big serving of one food. For example, it would take four to five eggs to reach your 30-40g protein target (one egg contains around seven grams of protein). Instead, you could have three eggs (21 grams of protein) plus a scoop of collagen powder in your spearmint tea or a smoothie with a scoop of protein powder as a drink on the side.

If, like many PCOS Cysters, you have spent much of your life following restrictive diets, eating a large breakfast can feel really overwhelming at first. I encourage you to stick with it and trust the process. This change will have a powerful impact on your PCOS within weeks.

You won't need to eat this much protein at other meals of the day. We will cover specific strategies for your lunch, dinner, and snacks once we have identified your PCOS root cause. I suggest sticking with this breakfast step for at least two to three weeks before moving on to making your next change. Taking the time to get used to this new habit will help you avoid getting overwhelmed by making too many changes at once.

By starting with improving your breakfast, you will notice that, for the rest of the day, you have increased energy, feel more full and satisfied, and have fewer cravings. This will make implementing the next change so much easier.

<u>Low sugar fruits to enjoy at breakfast time:</u>

The following fruits contain less than 7g of sugar per serve and are high in fiber and antioxidants, so are a great choice at breakfast time. Choose one of the following choices in the portion size listed (or smaller) to keep your blood sugar and insulin stable.

- ½ cup blackberries (6.2g sugar)
- ½ cup blueberries (6.8g sugar)
- 1 cup raspberries (6.5g sugar)
- 1 cup frozen mixed berries (6.5g sugar)
- 8 medium strawberries (3.8g sugar)

- 1 green kiwifruit (6.9g sugar)
- ½ grapefruit (6.2g sugar)
- ½ cup papaya (5g sugar)
- 1 apricot (3.8g sugar)
- 1 plum (4.3g sugar)

Summary: the PCOS Repair Breakfast principles:

- 30-40g protein
- No grains, starchy vegetables, legumes, or beans (e.g. chickpeas, baked beans) - tofu is allowed
- Unlimited non-starchy vegetables (e.g. zucchini, cauliflower, greens)
- Only the low-sugar fruits listed above, avoid other fruits
- No sugar or sweeteners (honey, maple syrup, sugar in your tea)
- Add some healthy fats (e.g. nut butter, coconut milk, avocado)

In your PCOS-Friendly Food Formula bonus resource, I've explained how to calculate the protein content of different breakfast foods. I've also included some of my favorite breakfast recipes that meet the PCOS Repair Breakfast principles to help get you started. To access your bonuses, go to nourishednaturalhealth.com/resources

FAQs about the PCOS Repair Breakfast

Can I use protein powder?

Yes!

I encourage you to go for whole food sources of protein where you can, but as a busy mum myself, I know how difficult finding time to make a large breakfast can be. If you would like to use a protein powder to meet your protein goals, look for one that is made from pea, egg white, collagen, hemp, beef protein isolate, or a combination of these.

Avoid protein powders that are made from whey as dairy products tend to stimulate insulin production. Look for a brand which uses natural sweeteners like stevia or monkfruit, and avoid artificial sweeteners like aspartame and sucralose.

Finally, check the nutrition facts label and look for a protein powder that contains less than 4 grams of carbohydrates per serve. Look for a flavor that you know you will enjoy, so that you will actually use your protein. Some companies offer trial sizes of different flavors so you can sample a few and find one that you really enjoy, before committing to buying a big tub.

I'm missing my regular breakfast. What are some swaps for my favorite breakfast foods?

It can be really hard to give up old favorites! Here are some of my favorite swaps:

- Swap oatmeal with banana for chia pudding (chia seeds soaked in almond or coconut milk) with a handful of berries
- Swap a banana smoothie (my old favorite breakfast) for a smoothie made with frozen zucchini or cauliflower, plus a flavored protein powder (e.g., vanilla or chocolate)

- Swap two eggs on regular toast for three eggs on a high protein/keto bread, or three eggs plus some smoked salmon or chicken sausage on a bed of sauteed greens
- Swap a cereal or muesli bowl with fruit and yogurt for bowl of coconut yogurt with a handful of nuts (like macadamias and walnuts) and fresh or frozen berries
- Swap a breakfast burrito made with a regular tortilla for a flaxseed wrap with a high protein filling like smoked salmon or bacon.

See your PCOS-Friendly Food Formula bonus resource for more recipe ideas.

Why shouldn't I skip breakfast or try intermittent fasting for my PCOS?

Intermittent fasting and skipping breakfast are commonly touted as "solutions" for women who are struggling with weight loss or other PCOS symptoms. However, the truth is, skipping breakfast is one of the worst things you can do for your hormone, blood sugar, and insulin levels.

Research shows that skipping breakfast has a far more significant impact on our hormones than skipping dinner.[22] An interesting study in 2013 took 60 women with PCOS and split them into two groups. The first group ate a large breakfast and a small dinner, and the second group ate a light breakfast and large dinner (similar to how many of us are used to eating).

Other than the timing of the meals, the women in both groups ate exactly the same ratios of carbs, fats, and proteins and the same calories over the course of the day. After 90 days, the women eating the large breakfast had a 50% decrease in testosterone levels, greatly improved insulin sensitivity, decreased androgenic symptoms, and a 50% increased ovulation rate.[22] The large dinner group had no changes.

This study suggests that something as simple as changing the timing of your meals could have a dramatic effect on your PCOS symptoms. PCOS causes our hormones to function differently than other women. This means that diets and styles of eating that work for other people might not work the same for us. It's important to keep this in mind.

How soon after waking should I eat my breakfast?

Ideally, aim to eat your breakfast within an hour of waking up. This is because the research shows this timing has the best effect on our blood sugar and insulin levels for the rest of the day. If you like to exercise first thing in the morning, you might like to have a small snack, and then eat a larger meal following the PCOS Repair Breakfast principles after you finish exercising. This is fine as well. After a few weeks of experimenting with this new way of eating, you'll find what works best for you.

What should I eat before working out in the morning?

Exercising first thing in the morning before eating can cause increased cortisol levels. I suggest having a small snack before starting your workout to prevent this. The best choice is a small carbohydrate plus protein or fat-rich snack. For example, half a banana with some almond or peanut butter.

Even though we are avoiding starch and sugar in the PCOS Repair Breakfast principles, if you eat this small amount of carbohydrates within 30 minutes of exercising, the carbs will be used as fuel for your workout and therefore won't contribute to significant insulin production. Once you have finished your workout, you can enjoy a larger meal following the high protein, low carb breakfast principles.

I'm feeling really full or unwell after eating such a large breakfast. Is this normal?

Many of my clients find they don't feel hungry in the morning and prefer to skip breakfast or have something light like some fruit or a piece of toast, only to be *starving* later in the day. For women with PCOS, our insulin issues, gut bacteria imbalances, and history of restriction and dieting can cause our hunger and fullness cues to be a little out of whack.

If you don't usually eat breakfast or are used to a lighter breakfast, it's normal for it to take time for your body to adjust. My clients have found that after two to three weeks, their hunger stabilizes and they feel much better eating this way. In the meantime, you might like to delay your lunch time meal or eat a smaller lunch until your hunger adjusts.

If you feel nauseous or struggle to eat first thing in the morning, try having one tablespoon of apple cider vinegar or lemon juice in a glass of water around ten minutes before your meal. This helps to stimulate appetite and prepare your stomach for food.

If you struggle to eat a full breakfast, try a drinkable breakfast like a smoothie that still meets the PCOS Repair Breakfast principles. You could try sipping on this over a longer period of time as you go about your morning routine.

Remember, you likely won't have to eat this much protein at breakfast forever, just while your insulin and other hormones are finding balance again, which usually takes around three months.

I'm feeling hungry two hours after eating this breakfast. Is this normal?

If you are feeling hungry within two hours despite hitting the 30-40 grams of protein target, try adding some extra healthy fats to your breakfast to keep you fuller for longer. Ideally, this breakfast should keep you full for at least three to four hours. My favorite healthy fats are coconut milk (great in smoothies), nut butter, avocado, and olive oil.

What about dairy?

We'll cover whether or not reducing dairy could be helpful for your type PCOS in chapter 17, however as a general rule, dairy tends to cause an increase in insulin, so it's best minimized at breakfast time. You can swap dairy for coconut or almond milks and yogurts.

How do I know if a vegetable is low in starch?

A good rule of thumb is vegetables that grow above the ground are generally lower in starch and higher in fiber. Vegetables that grow below the ground tend to be starchy vegetables (with the exception of onion and garlic). To find out if a particular vegetable is low or high in starch, you can Google "is [insert vegetable] a starchy vegetable?". This tends to be a pretty accurate way of determining it.

Some of the most common starchy vegetables to avoid in your breakfast include potato, sweet potato, corn, beans and legumes, yams, peas, pumpkin, and butternut squash. You'll be able to enjoy these foods later on in the day.

Some of the most common non-starchy vegetables include asparagus, broccoli, Brussels sprouts, cabbage, cauliflower, cucumber, eggplant, mushrooms, onion, garlic, capsicum (peppers), spinach, kale, tomato, and zucchini. You can enjoy as much of these non-starchy vegetables as you like – there is no limit as they won't cause a spike in your blood sugar.

For more ideas on foods to include in your PCOS Repair Breakfast, see your bonus resource PCOS-Friendly Food Formula.

ACTION STEP:

Post a photo of your PCOS Repair Breakfast in the Cysterhood community. If you haven't joined our community, head to nourishednaturalhealth.com/resources to sign up for free.

Chapter 6

PCOS Superfoods

Once you get the hang of your PCOS Repair breakfast and feel inspired to keep reducing your PCOS symptoms, check out some of the recommendations below for more things to *add* into your diet.

Many Cysters have spent years being told they need to lose weight to improve their PCOS. This means that we have often spent a long time following restrictive diets, cutting things out of our lives, and feeling deprived. My approach to managing your PCOS is different.

> "Instead of focussing on things to go *without*, I want you to focus on all of the incredibly helpful things you can *add in*."

This simple mindset shift from restriction to abundance has a powerful impact on your ability to stick to the changes we'll cover in the rest of this book. By eating *more* of the things that are helpful for PCOS, you will not only be able to recover your relationship with food, but you will also naturally crowd out less helpful foods without ever feeling deprived.

While my number one goal for you after reading this book is to be free of your symptoms and thrive with PCOS, I also want you to have fun and enjoy the process! I go into depth about each of these foods plus fun tips and tricks to enjoy them in my *14 Day Fast Start Challenge*. If you haven't already, join the challenge at pcosrepair.com/challenge

The list below is by no means a list of foods that *must* be eaten to heal your PCOS. It is simply a guide to nutritious foods that you may want to consider adding to your current diet to boost your results. These foods are helpful no matter which type of PCOS you have.

SPOTLIGHT: Jaime's story - losing weight whilst feeling full and satisfied

Jaime and I started working together three months after she was diagnosed with PCOS due to her missing periods and inability to lose weight. She wasn't able to have a natural period without the use of medication. Like so many other Cysters, she was told by her doctor she needed to exercise more, lose weight and come back when she was ready to get pregnant. This advice left her feeling completely lost and disheartened. She'd tried dieting in the past with no results and felt overwhelmed at having to go on yet another restrictive meal plan.

Jaime told me that her visits to her doctor had always been rushed. She felt like no one had taken the time to explain to her what was going on with her body, which made sticking to changes really difficult. Before making any tweaks to her diet and lifestyle, we started by simply exploring what PCOS was and how this hormonal imbalance was contributing to her symptoms.

Empowered with the knowledge about what her body needed to thrive, we then addressed her reliance on coffee and sugar which she felt were 'ruling her life'. We explored how these foods were contributing to her PCOS and swapped them for alternatives like decaf green tea and natural sweeteners.

We filled her plate with nourishing, PCOS-friendly foods (like those covered in this chapter) so that she felt full and satiated after all her meals. Jaime loved that she could eat freely and enjoy herself (a stark contrast to the restrictive diets she had tried in the past!). Meditation and journaling also became integral parts of her PCOS repair toolkit and she found that supporting her emotional health was just as important as her physical health.

Over the next three months, Jaime lost 20 pounds (9 kilograms) without ever feeling deprived. Her period started to arrive regularly, without using medication and she finally felt in control of her PCOS. You can listen to Jaime's full story at nourishednaturalhealth.com/resources

Flax Seeds

Flax seeds contain a compound called lignan that can reduce 5-alpha reductase – the enzyme responsible for converting testosterone into its super-potent cousin, DHT.[23] Studies suggest adding flaxseeds to your daily meals is an effective way to support healthy androgen levels.[24]

Flax seeds are best eaten ground rather than whole as the fibrous husks are very difficult to digest. Try grinding whole seeds in a coffee or spice grinder, or buy them pre-ground and store in the fridge.

I suggest one to two tablespoons daily. If these are a new food for you or you don't consume much fiber, start slow (around a ½ tablespoon daily) and gradually work your way up to two tablespoons to reduce any possible digestive discomfort. My favorite way to enjoy ground flaxseeds is by adding a big scoop into my morning PCOS Repair Chocolate Thickshake (you'll find this recipe in your PCOS-Friendly Food Formula bonus).

Brazil nuts

The top source of selenium, the humble Brazil nut is a great way of naturally supporting your thyroid. Your thyroid gland has the highest concentration of selenium of any organ in your body and requires sufficient levels to keep your thyroid hormones in balance.

Research shows that women with PCOS are three times more likely to suffer from thyroid disorders like Hashimoto's thyroiditis.[25] Imbalances in thyroid hormones contribute to worsened PCOS symptoms, irregular ovulation, weight gain, infertility, and insulin resistance.[26] For more information on how to support your thyroid, see chapter 16.

Just two to three Brazil nuts daily is enough to meet your selenium needs. Consuming more than this can easily put you at a toxic level of selenium, so go easy on these nuts! Snacking on a couple of Brazil nuts each day is a great way to support your thyroid and is safe even if you have existing issues with your thyroid.

Apple Cider Vinegar

Apple cider vinegar has been shown to reduce fasting blood sugar levels and improve insulin resistance.[27] It also helps to stimulate your appetite and support healthy weight loss by improving your gut bacteria.[28] It is a great choice if you feel nauseous or don't have an appetite in the morning.

I like to start my day with a tablespoon of apple cider vinegar in a small glass of water around ten minutes before my breakfast as I find this helps to boost my appetite and improve my digestion. If this is new for you, start with a teaspoon and work your way up to a tablespoon. If you notice any heartburn or digestive discomfort, reduce your amount until you find the right dose for you.

Green tea

Green tea has been shown to support PCOS symptoms by improving how well your body handles glucose, as well as supporting healthy weight loss.[29] Like spearmint tea, green tea also has androgen-lowering effects.[30]

Ideally, opt for decaf green tea because some types of PCOS benefit from a reduction in caffeine, particularly if you relate to the Adrenal PCOS type. (More on this in chapter 14).

Cinnamon

Cinnamon is one of the best natural insulin sensitizing spices. A 2007 study gave women with PCOS either cinnamon or a placebo daily for eight weeks.[31] After two months, the women consuming cinnamon had a significant reduction in insulin resistance, whereas there was no change in the placebo group. Another 2021 study found that cinnamon greatly improved HOMA-IR scores (an accurate measurement of insulin) and caused no side effects.[32]

As little as two teaspoons of ground cinnamon daily can improve insulin sensitivity, the root cause of at least 80% of PCOS cases. Try sprinkling some cinnamon over your breakfast, adding it to a smoothie, mixing it into a homemade protein ball, or even baking it on pumpkin or sweet potato.

Turmeric

Turmeric contains a powerful anti-inflammatory compound called curcumin. Women with PCOS have been shown to have higher levels of inflammation, sometimes to the extent that it's the number one root cause of your PCOS (more on this in chapter 16).

Curcumin has been shown to improve fasting glucose, fasting insulin, HOMA-IR, and cholesterol levels in women with PCOS.[33] More research is needed to determine the exact dosages and forms of turmeric that are best, however adding some turmeric powder to your cooking is a safe and easy way to reduce your inflammation and improve your PCOS symptoms.

Fermented foods

We've known for a long time that women with PCOS have different gut microbiomes to other women.[34] Research shows that certain gut bacteria can cause insulin resistance, hyperandrogenism, chronic inflammation, obesity, and diabetes – all key features in PCOS.[34]

Supporting your gut microbiome balance is key in managing PCOS, particularly if you suffer from digestive issues alongside your PCOS symptoms. I've covered specific gut health strategies for you in your bonus resource Beat The Bloat, but for now, adding some fermented foods into your diet is a great way to support your gut.

My favorite fermented foods to include are sauerkraut, kimchi, kombucha, and coconut kefir. If you are new to eating these foods, add them into your diet slowly as large amounts can initially cause some digestive discomfort. This will usually pass after a few weeks of including these foods.

Oily fish

Oily fish like salmon, sardines, and mackerel contain high amounts of omega-3 fatty acid - a naturally anti-inflammatory healthy fat source. Studies show that omega-3 supplementation improves insulin resistance and reduces the risk of developing type 2 diabetes.[35]

Omega-3 also helps to reduce acne by lowering inflammation in your skin,[36] so is a great way to tackle this common PCOS symptom while you work on your root cause.

Aim to enjoy oily fish three to four times per week to gain the benefits. If you struggle to meet this intake or for faster results, consider a high-quality Omega 3 supplement like Nourished Daily Omega+.

Berries

Dark berries like blueberries, raspberries, and blackberries contain high levels of antioxidants – compounds that naturally fight oxidative stress and help to lower inflammation in your body. Women with PCOS have been shown to have higher levels of oxidative stress[37] and this can be reduced by eating a diet rich in antioxidants. This is particularly true if you are dealing with Inflammatory PCOS – one of the four types of PCOS we will cover in chapter 16.

Berries are also low in sugar compared to most other fruits, meaning they won't spike your blood sugar levels as significantly. They are a great choice to satisfy your sugar cravings while keeping your insulin levels in check. I love adding ½ to 1 cup of frozen berries to my morning smoothie, or enjoying fresh berries with some coconut yogurt as a snack.

ACTION STEP:

Which one of these foods are you going to add into your meals? Tell us in the PCOS Repair Cysterhood community and share how you're eating it! If you haven't joined our community, head to nourishednaturalhealth.com/resources to sign up for free.

STEP TWO: Identify Your Root Cause

Now that you have switched your breakfast and addressed your body's overproduction of androgens, you are probably noticing some small but significant changes. More energy in the mornings? Better sleep? Clearer skin? Less sugar cravings? Or maybe fewer hangry attacks?

Reducing your androgen levels will go a long way in improving your symptoms; however, to truly heal your PCOS, we need to dig deeper and uncover your unique PCOS root cause. This section will help you understand the four most common root causes of PCOS and how to work out which one (or combination) you are. We will then create an individualized plan to address your unique root cause in the next section.

I first heard of the idea of PCOS types from Naturopathic Doctor Lara Briden in her revolutionary 2018 book *The Period Repair Manual.*[38] In her book, she outlines the four "functional subtypes" of PCOS that she has observed in her clinical practice. Since then, researchers have gone on to confirm the existence of different underlying biological mechanisms that drive PCOS and expressed the need to individualize treatment for each.[7]

When I started applying this knowledge in my own practice, I immediately saw incredible results. As outlined previously, the four root causes of PCOS are insulin resistance, stress, coming off hormonal birth control, and inflammation. Neglecting these distinct differences in PCOS cases is what prevents so many women from getting the right treatment to heal their PCOS for good.

Most women with PCOS have a combination of two or three root causes, particularly if your primary root cause has been unaddressed for a long time. This is because when one body system is out of balance, it can trigger others to suffer too.

For example, if your primary root cause is high stress hormones (Adrenal PCOS), you will be making extra cortisol (our main stress hormone). Cortisol triggers your body to dump extra glucose into your blood to help you fight or run from danger. Over time, if you don't address the high cortisol, the extra glucose in your blood can lead to insulin resistance.

In this scenario, tackling your stress hormones first will help to improve insulin resistance. For each PCOS case, there tends to be a primary root cause that is having the biggest impact on our symptoms. Fixing this will have a ripple effect, knocking down all of your other symptoms.

If you find that multiple root causes apply to you after reading this section, pick the one that feels most impactful to you and start there. You can always add on some extra support from the other sections of this book once you have worked through your primary root cause. If you aren't sure about your primary root cause and need help, my team and I am here for you in the PCOS Repair Cysterhood community. Go to nourishednaturalhealth.com/resources to join our free community if you haven't done so already.

To work out your primary root cause, we will look at the signs and symptoms of each of the four types. If you wish, you can also add in some testing to confirm your root cause. I'll outline the best tests for each root cause in this chapter if you decide to pursue this. However, in most cases, your hunger, sugar cravings, weight distribution, stress levels, sleep, and other symptoms can tell us a huge amount about what is contributing to your PCOS.

Chapter 7

Insulin-Resistant PCOS (Type 1)

This is by far the most common root cause of PCOS. At least 80% of Cysters have some level of insulin resistance,[39] including those who don't have excess body weight (often referred to as "lean PCOS"). Weight gain is only one symptom of insulin resistance, and it doesn't happen for all Insulin-Resistant PCOS Cysters. If you've been told you don't have a problem with insulin because you're not overweight, you might be missing out on the correct treatment for your PCOS.

When researchers used the most sensitive insulin resistance tests to compare women with and without PCOS (controls), they found an interesting difference.[40] 75% of lean women with PCOS had insulin resistance compared with only 24% of lean women controls. The same study found insulin resistance in 95% of overweight women with PCOS, compared with only 62% of overweight controls.

This study reveals that the insulin resistance associated with PCOS is independent of weight gain. In other words, *weight gain isn't the cause of insulin resistance in PCOS*. In fact, the opposite is true – insulin resistance is often the cause of weight gain. If you aren't overweight, there is still a significant chance that insulin resistance is driving your symptoms. PCOS significantly increases our chances of having issues with insulin, regardless of weight.

My PCOS fertility journey

Unfortunately, the fact that you can have insulin resistance without weight gain in PCOS isn't common knowledge. Many doctors believe that if you have PCOS and don't have weight gain as a symptom, there is nothing that you can do. I experienced this first hand when I began my PCOS fertility journey.

I visited my doctor, excited to get my body ready to try for a baby in the next few months. I asked her what I could do to support my hormones and increase my chances of falling pregnant naturally. By this point, I had been working on my PCOS for years and had achieved a healthy weight and clear skin, but my cycles were still a little wonky.

I was told that because I wasn't overweight there was nothing else I could do naturally. I left with a referral in my hand to a fertility specialist and the advice that I would probably need fertility drugs to fall pregnant. We hadn't even started trying for a baby yet! I was crushingly disappointed to hear the road ahead would be so difficult.

Fast forward nine months, and that referral sat unopened on my desk. I had improved my insulin and stress hormones naturally, regulated my cycle and was six weeks pregnant after three months of trying naturally.

This isn't to say that fertility drugs aren't helpful or necessary in some cases. However, all too often I have seen women pushed down this path before working on some of the most basic lifestyle factors like what you eat, how you move, and how you manage stress.

If you have received the same advice as I did, I urge you to dedicate the next six months to implementing the advice in this book first. Even if you don't fall pregnant naturally, you will have significantly higher success rates with fertility interventions and an easier, healthier pregnancy and baby.

How insulin resistance causes PCOS symptoms

Remember the taxi driver analogy from chapter two? Insulin resistance happens when our cells become "deaf" to the signals of insulin telling them to open up and let sugar from our blood inside for storage. Insulin is like a key that fits into the lock on the cell door. In insulin resistance, this key has become a little rusty, and it takes a lot of fiddling to get the door open.

This extra time taken to open the cell door means that insulin stays raised in the blood for a lot longer than it should. If you have high levels of insulin for a long time, it triggers your ovaries to start producing extra testosterone and other androgens.

Excess insulin also lowers an important protein called sex hormone binding globulin (SHBG). I like to think of SHBG as a hormone sponge. Its main role is to mop up excess hormones and keep levels balanced. When you have higher levels of androgens floating around, *combined* with lower SHBG, it's a recipe for disaster.

Instead of being mopped up, the androgens run free and get into your scalp hair follicles, killing them and making them fall out. They get into the pores in your skin, clogging them and causing acne. And they get into your face and chest hair follicles and change your unnoticeable baby hairs into thick, coarse, black hairs. To make matters worse, high testosterone levels trigger even more insulin production, creating a frustrating spiral where androgen levels continue to rise.[41]

High insulin also causes your brain to secrete less follicle stimulating hormone (FSH). FSH is needed to trigger your follicles (baby eggs) to grow to the right size needed for you to ovulate. Without enough FSH, you either fail to ovulate altogether (meaning your period disappears) or it takes much longer to ovulate (causing very long gaps between periods).[42]

Finally, high insulin levels cause another key hormone involved with ovulation, luteinizing hormone (LH), to be secreted in high levels. In the right amounts, LH is needed to trigger ovulation. When levels are too high, your body shuts down or delays ovulation, further contributing to missing or irregular periods.[42]

Signs and Symptoms of Insulin Resistance

Take the quiz below to rate the likelihood of insulin being a root cause of your PCOS. Each time you answer yes, give yourself one point.

- ☐ I have dark, velvety patches in the folds of my skin (acanthosis nigricans)
- ☐ I crave sweets/sugar during the day
- ☐ I feel tired after meals
- ☐ I am very hungry if I haven't eaten for three hours (or I feel angry, jittery or brain foggy when I haven't eaten)
- ☐ I feel like I always need something sweet after finishing a meal (even when I'm full)
- ☐ I crave stimulants like coffee after a meal
- ☐ I have skin tags
- ☐ I easily put on weight around my midsection or struggle to lose weight in this area
- ☐ I have a family history of diabetes or pre-diabetes
- ☐ Waist circumference greater than 80cm (32 inches) → *see below for more info*
- ☐ I have been told I am pre-diabetic, or I have high fasting insulin or glucose on blood tests

If you said yes to **four or more of the points above**, there's a high chance insulin resistance is the root cause of your PCOS. If you aren't sure or would like to confirm this with testing, see below for the best tests to diagnose insulin resistance. Testing is optional. If it's not within your budget right now but you relate to the symptoms above, you can jump ahead to chapter 13 and start implementing the Insulin-Resistant PCOS protocol.

Problems with Common Tests for Insulin Resistance

You might not know if you have insulin resistance because your doctor didn't order the most sensitive tests. The most commonly used tests are fasting glucose and HbA1C. These tests are unfortunately not sensitive enough to pick up on early stage insulin resistance, and are better at diagnosing severe insulin resistance like that in type 2 diabetes.

A 2014 study found that HbA1C missed 45% of people with type 2 diabetes,[43] which is a more severe form of insulin resistance. This means that this test has a high likelihood of missing early stage insulin resistance.

Fasting blood glucose is another commonly used test, however the upper "normal" limits set by most pathology laboratories are likely far too high. The commonly accepted upper limit for fasting blood glucose is 100mg/dL (meaning that a number below 100 is considered normal). A 2005 study showed that people with fasting blood glucose levels between 91-99mg/dL went on to develop type 2 diabetes.[44]

If you've ever had an oral glucose tolerance test before (OGTT), you likely haven't forgotten it! This test involves drinking a sickly sweet drink and having your blood taken every hour for two to three hours to measure the rise and fall in your glucose levels. It's commonly used in pregnancy to diagnose gestational diabetes.

Whilst more accurate than the two previous tests, an OGTT also won't pick up the early stages of insulin resistance because it measures glucose rather than insulin. An interesting study showed that OGTTs missed up to 50% of people with diabetes.[45]

The reason that blood glucose is often normal in insulin resistance is because your insulin is being secreted at incredibly high amounts in order to keep glucose low. This means that when all we look at is your glucose levels, they appear normal. However, behind the scenes, your insulin is working overtime to keep glucose balanced. Only testing glucose means you could miss out on the correct diagnosis and treatment for your PCOS.

If your doctor has ruled out insulin resistance by testing your fasting blood glucose, HbA1C, or OGTT and you feel it could still be an issue for you, don't be afraid to ask for further testing. I've covered the best tests to ask for below.

Gold Standard Tests for Insulin Resistance

Blood Test

The most accurate test for insulin resistance is a *Glucose Tolerance with Insulin Assay*. This is similar to an OGTT, but measures insulin as well as glucose. You will have your blood taken fasting and then at one and two hour intervals after drinking a glucose drink. This test has been shown to be 75% more effective at detecting diabetes and pre-diabetes than the traditional OGTT.[46]

Ideally, your fasting insulin should be less than 10mlU/L (60pmol/L). At the one- and two-hour marks after your sugar drink, your insulin should be less than 60mlU/L (410pmol/L). If it's higher than this, it indicates insulin resistance is a problem for you.

This test is far less common than a standard OGTT, fasting glucose, or HbA1C, so don't be surprised if your doctor hasn't heard of it. Keep asking or find a new practitioner who can support you to get access to the right testing to rule in or out insulin resistance.

Measure Your Waist

Insulin resistance can cause weight to be deposited around your midsection. The higher your waist circumference is, the more likely you are to have insulin resistance.

Grab out your tape measure and place it at the top of your hip bone. Then bring the tape measure around your body in line with your belly button. Make sure it's straight and even. Take a breath in and out and relax your belly (make sure you're not holding it in).

Check the number on the tape measure. For women, a measurement of 80cm (32 inches) indicates a higher likelihood of insulin resistance. The risk increases the further above 80cm your waist measurement is.

Remember that there is a misconception that being overweight *causes* insulin resistance. This means that you don't have to have a high waist measurement or be overweight to have insulin resistance – it just increases your chances. The signs and symptoms listed above also give us a clear indication of whether insulin is a problem for you.

Metformin

If you are overweight or have been diagnosed with insulin resistance, there's a good chance you've been offered Metformin – the leading insulin-sensitizing drug. Metformin helps to improve your body's sensitivity to insulin and can be really helpful in treating this root cause for some women.

Unfortunately, this drug is associated with a high rate of side effects – more than 50% of women report gastrointestinal side effects (nausea, diarrhea, and vomiting).[47] Metformin is also well known to cause vitamin B12 deficiency, so if you are using this drug to manage your insulin levels, I highly recommend a daily B12 supplement to combat this.

Whether or not to use Metformin for your PCOS is a personal choice. You can achieve the same results – if not better – as Metformin by following the diet and lifestyle changes in this book. If you are noticing side effects from Metformin and would like to try an alternative, inositol has been shown head-to-head against Metformin to achieve higher success in weight loss, restoring regular ovulation and natural pregnancy, without the side effects.[21] I recommend Nourished Cycle Regulate + Ovulate as it contains the ideal 40:1 ratio of myo-inositol and D-chiroinositol. You can purchase Cycle Regulate + Ovulate via nourishednaturalhealth.com/resources

> *Changing what you eat, how you move and which supplements you take is the most effective way to reverse insulin resistance and thrive with PCOS.*

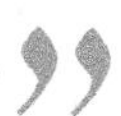

SPOTLIGHT: Maria's intense sugar cravings

Maria joined my group program in 2019 after struggling with lean PCOS for most of her life. A few weeks into the program, Maria reached out to me, incredulous. We had just covered how eating a diet high in sugar can trigger insulin resistance and a light bulb had gone off for her. Maria had always thought about food as something for pleasure. Because she didn't deal with weight gain as a symptom of her PCOS, she had never considered the importance of what she was eating. She ate pastries and bread every day, had a self proclaimed sweet tooth, and rarely ever ate vegetables. She told me "in all the years that I've had PCOS, no one ever told me that food could be impacting my symptoms!". Over the next few weeks, we made some simple tweaks to how Maria created her meals, and before long her reliance on sugar disappeared. Her cycle regulated and her hair stopped falling out. Maria now knows she doesn't need sugar for energy and can choose to enjoy pastries on special occasions without feeling out of control. Watch Maria's story via nourishednaturalhealth.com/resources

What causes insulin resistance?

Developing insulin resistance is usually a combination of your genetics (being "predisposed") and your environment (what you eat, how you move, sleep, and stress). Similar to the way that we end up with PCOS, you are probably born with a higher likelihood of developing insulin resistance – this is why you saw a family history of diabetes or pre-diabetes as one of the quiz questions earlier in this chapter.

Just having a family history or genetic predisposition doesn't necessarily mean you will end up with insulin resistance, however. It's how you eat, move, sleep, manage stress, and many other factors in your environment that switch on this condition. For example, a diet high in fructose (a type of sugar) has been shown to increase the risk.[48] Sleep quality is another risk factor. Just a single night of sleep deprivation has been shown to reduce insulin sensitivity the following day,[49] and chronic sleep deprivation increases the risk of developing lasting insulin resistance.

Not exercising regularly is another area researchers are exploring[50] as movement helps to sensitize your muscles to insulin. Your mother's pregnancy with you might also be a factor. Researchers are finding links between mothers who experienced a major stressful life event during pregnancy and their adult children's risk of developing insulin resistance, even without a family history of diabetes.[51] If your mother had gestational diabetes during her pregnancy with you, your risk also increases for insulin resistance later in life.[52] Even your gut bacteria play a role in your sensitivity to insulin and improving gut health can reduce insulin resistance.[53]

While we can't change your genetics or your mother's pregnancy with you, there is so much we *can* do to tweak the other environmental factors in your favor. Simple changes to your meals, exercise, mindfulness, sleep, gut health, and supplement regime can be foundational in reversing your insulin resistance. In the next section of the book, we'll cover the most impactful changes you can make to support this root cause so you can thrive with PCOS.

ACTION STEP:

Is Insulin Resistance your PCOS type? Tell us in the PCOS Repair Cysterhood community and connect with other Type 1 Cysters! Go to nourishednaturalhealth.com/resources if you haven't already joined our free community.

Chapter 8

Adrenal PCOS (Type 2)

The second most common type of PCOS is caused by high levels of stress hormones. In the last section, we learned that excess insulin causes your ovaries to produce higher amounts of testosterone. This is the most common root cause of PCOS and accounts for at least 80% of PCOS cases.

In adrenal PCOS, the problem isn't in your ovaries but in your adrenal glands. High levels of stress triggers your brain to secrete adrenocorticotropic hormone (ACTH). The ACTH triggers your adrenal glands to secrete cortisol, adrenaline, and another hormone called dehydroepiandrosterone sulfate (DHEAS) to help us respond to stress or danger. When stress continues for a long time, both cortisol and DHEAS levels continue to rise, leading to Adrenal PCOS.

DHEAS is a member of the androgen family, like testosterone, and causes very similar symptoms like acne, hair loss, and hair growth. Research shows that at least 20-30% of women with PCOS have adrenal androgen excess.[54] While the research in this area is still in its infancy, several studies suggest there may be a genetic link between women with adrenal androgen excess,[54] meaning certain Cysters are more likely to develop this form of PCOS.

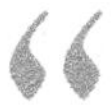 Adrenal PCOS is essentially an abnormal response to stress. 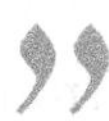

You might experience a similar amount of stress to your friend or partner, but find that while they can carry on relatively unscathed, your PCOS symptoms flare up like they're going out of fashion.

How does DHEAS cause PCOS symptoms?

DHEAS functions very similarly in the body to testosterone. In the right amounts, both testosterone and DHEAS improve our sex drive, boost our mood and help us feel good. In excess, they get into your follicles, causing hair loss on your scalp, excess hair growth on your face, chest, and breasts, and acne on your face, chest, and back. Like testosterone, DHEAS is also converted to DHT, increasing the potency and intensity of your androgenic symptoms (read back over chapter 2 for a refresher).

DHEAS gets into your ovaries and affects the quality of your eggs.[55] In some cases, it can affect the release of LH from your brain, which causes halted or delayed ovulation. This is why you might experience very long gaps between your periods and have issues falling pregnant.

Interestingly, Adrenal PCOS doesn't contribute to weight gain in the same way as insulin resistance, so if you don't suffer from weight gain as a symptom, you may be more likely to be dealing with Adrenal

PCOS.[56] You can still have Adrenal PCOS if you are overweight, but it is more likely if you have lean PCOS.

If your main symptoms are acne and hair changes, you don't suffer from weight gain and you have normal testosterone results on your blood tests, there's a good chance you fit the Adrenal PCOS picture.

DHEAS causes many of the same symptoms as high testosterone but is not commonly measured by doctors despite its prevalence. I have worked with a huge number of confused clients who are experiencing all the symptoms of androgen excess, but have been told by their doctor that their testosterone levels are normal (or even low). If this is you, remember that there are other androgens like DHEAS that can cause the same symptoms as high testosterone that may not have been measured on your blood tests.

What causes high stress hormones?

When I mention "stress" I have likely conjured up an image in your mind of the overworked business woman with an overflowing inbox and looming deadlines. Or maybe an exhausted mother stuck in traffic with screaming children in the backseat.

The reality is there are many "stressors" that can trigger this increased production of cortisol and DHEAS. Psychological stress like that described in the scenarios above is very real in our modern world and absolutely contributes to stress hormone production.

However, other areas you may not have considered that could be contributing to your PCOS symptoms include: poor sleep, chronic infections, loneliness, restrictive dieting, over-exercising, autoimmune disease, and over-consumption of stimulants like caffeine.

Even if you don't feel "stressed out," you may be hypersensitive to a regular level of stress hormones. In the opening chapter of this book, we looked at an interesting study that showed that stress experienced during puberty can contribute to the development of PCOS later in life.

Dealing with higher levels of stress in this critical development window likely "hardwires" your brain to be overly sensitive to the effects of stress later in life. This might be relevant to you if you had a significant loss or traumatic event occur during adolescence, or engaged in extreme dieting or exercise at this time.

A Personal Story – Adrenal PCOS was my missing link

Adrenal PCOS was the missing link that tied all of my symptoms together after years of struggling. Five years into my PCOS journey, I was following an insulin-resistant way of eating and was noticing massive changes to my sugar cravings, moods, and energy. My skin was starting to clear, but my cycles were still arriving every 60-70 days. I was frustrated because I had been working so hard on my health whilst also juggling two jobs, university study, and trying to keep up some semblance of a social life.

I visited my doctor for more advice and she suggested we test my testosterone levels. A week later, she called me to tell me my levels were completely normal and she didn't know why my cycles were still so irregular.

I knew there were other androgens that could be contributing to my symptoms, so I took a urine test to measure my DHEAS and cortisol. To my suprise, my DHEAS levels came back through the roof! My cortisol levels were also well out of range. These tests showed I had been much more stressed out than I realized.

This was a huge wakeup call to the impact of stress on my PCOS symptoms. I was getting up at 5am every morning to do a HIIT workout because I knew this improved insulin, then heading off to work followed by night classes at university and weekends packed full of social engagements. I was strictly following a low carb style of eating and I was pushing myself to do more and be more perfect in every area of my life.

It wasn't until I pulled back on my own expectations of myself that my symptoms finally resolved. I switched some of my workouts to slow walks or swims at the beach. I added a ten minute morning meditation to start the day with lowered stress hormones. I started saying "No" to events and engagements that didn't light me up and adopted an 80/20 approach to my way of eating (more on this in chapter 22).

After three months of taking this more relaxed approach, my cycles shortened to 32 days and my skin completely cleared. I had finally found the missing piece to heal my PCOS at the core.

Even though the HIIT workouts and strict way of eating were helping my insulin, following them 100% was contributing to more stress hormones and therefore more DHEAS. I had to find a balance that kept both my cortisol and insulin in check at the same time. At the end of this chapter, we'll look at how to manage multiple root causes at the same time.

Common signs and symptoms of Adrenal PCOS

Take the quiz below to rate the likelihood of high stress hormones being a root cause of your PCOS. Each time you answer yes, give yourself one point.

- ☐ I scored less than four on the Insulin Resistance quiz (or I have ruled out insulin resistance with testing)
- ☐ I have experienced a high amount of stress in the last five years
- ☐ I feel that I react strongly to stressful situations or it takes me a long time to recover
- ☐ I experienced significant stress or a major life event during puberty (e.g., loss of a loved one) or I engaged in extreme dieting at this time
- ☐ I have normal (or low) testosterone or androstenedione levels on blood tests, but still have androgenic symptoms (acne, hair loss on my head, thick/dark hair growth on my body)
- ☐ I have high DHEAS levels on blood or urine tests
- ☐ I often find I have my best energy after 6pm (or before bed)
- ☐ I struggle to get up and going in the morning

- ☐ I rely on caffeine or other stimulants for energy
- ☐ I wake up tired even after seven hours of sleep
- ☐ I do more than six hours of medium to high intensity exercise per week (e.g., running, HIIT, cross fit, boxing)
- ☐ I get headaches when I am stressed or exhausted
- ☐ Weight gain isn't one of my symptoms

If you said yes to six or more of the points above, there's a high chance stress hormones are a driving force behind your PCOS. If you aren't sure or would like to confirm this with testing, see below for the best tests to confirm this. Testing is optional and if it's not within your budget right now, but you relate to the symptoms above, you can jump ahead to chapter 14 and start implementing the Adrenal PCOS protocol.

What if I have high scores for Insulin Resistance and Adrenal PCOS?

One of the most common PCOS types is a combination of Insulin Resistance and Adrenal (type 1 + 2). This is because high stress hormones increase insulin resistance. Insulin resistance puts stress on your body, worsening adrenal PCOS.

As you can see, both conditions contribute to each other. While this might feel overwhelming at first, it is actually a positive situation because it means that no matter which root cause you start tackling first, the other will respond positively as well.

If you relate strongly to both types, I suggest starting with the Insulin Resistance Core Treatment Protocol in the next section of the book.

Once you feel confident with this, you can move onto the Adrenal Core Treatment Protocol and slowly build in some of these aspects to your existing habits.

If you would prefer to start with Adrenal and then move onto Insulin Resistance because you feel stress is a bigger issue for you right now, that's completely fine as well. Both protocols will work in either order, and you will find several overlaps between them.

Testing to confirm Adrenal PCOS

The best test to confirm Adrenal PCOS is a blood or urine test measuring DHEAS.

You can test your blood cortisol, however this hormone is difficult to measure accurately in a standard blood test. If you are curious, **salivary or urinary cortisol and cortisone** (a breakdown product of cortisol) are more sensitive tests that can pick up earlier changes. These two hormones can be tested at the same time and are best measured several times over the course of a day. Doing so allows you to see this rise and fall of your stress hormones and DHEAS and provides great insight into Adrenal PCOS.

These tests are best accessed through a practitioner who is trained in ordering and interpreting the Dried Urine Test for Comprehensive Hormones (DUTCH). You can find a list of accredited practitioners at https://dutchtest.com/find-a-dutch-provider/. Please note that these tests are not required to move ahead and start implementing the Adrenal PCOS Protocol – they simply provide interesting insight into how your body is managing stress and give you a reference point to compare with after making changes.

ACTION STEP:

Is Adrenal your PCOS type? Tell us in the PCOS Repair Cysterhood Community and connect with other Type 2 Cysters! Go to nourishednaturalhealth.com/resources if you haven't already joined our free community.

Chapter 9

Post-Pill PCOS (Type 3)

Have you recently come off hormonal birth control (HBC) and noticed your PCOS symptoms for the first time? It's common for certain types of birth control to trigger the symptoms of PCOS like acne, hair changes, and irregular cycles when you stop using them. The good news is these are usually *temporary.*

The key thing to understand about this root cause is that if you had the symptoms of PCOS *before* going on HBC, you don't have true Post-Pill PCOS. Coming off birth control can trigger your existing symptoms to flare up, however it didn't *cause* your PCOS. In this situation, we need to dig deeper and work out what was driving your PCOS *before* you took birth control.

It's common to be prescribed HBC *because* of the symptoms of PCOS. This is because the synthetic hormones can help to reduce acne and unwanted hair growth while you take HBC. HBC can also make you feel like you're having a regular bleed by shutting down your ovulation (jump back to chapter two for more on why the pill can't regulate your period).

If you were given HBC to help you deal with the symptoms of PCOS, they went away while you took HBC, but returned after you stopped, you *don't* have Post-Pill PCOS – you have a different root cause. HBC essentially masks the symptoms of PCOS by suppressing your natural hormone levels. See the other chapters in this section for more information on the other three types of PCOS to work out which one you have.

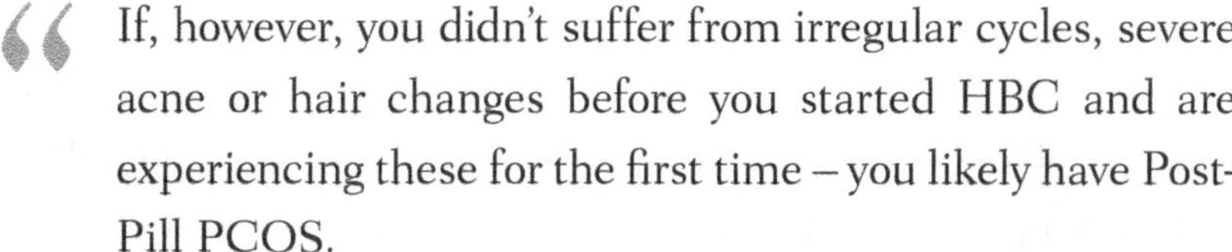

> "If, however, you didn't suffer from irregular cycles, severe acne or hair changes before you started HBC and are experiencing these for the first time – you likely have Post-Pill PCOS."

This PCOS type is caused by a withdrawal from the synthetic hormones in HBC. Some types of HBC are more likely to cause Post-Pill PCOS than others. The most common are birth control pills that contain drospirenone or cyproterone. Common brands of these pills include Yaz, Yasmin, Diane, and Brenda.

Unlike the other root causes of PCOS, this type is temporary and will likely resolve in 12 to 24 months. In the meantime, there is plenty we can do to suppress your body's overproduction of androgens and encourage your cycle to become regular again. We'll cover this in more detail in the next section.

How does HBC cause PCOS symptoms?

The reason certain types of HBC are so commonly prescribed for acne and hair growth is because they strongly suppress your body's production of sebum (skin oil). One study showed that cyproterone acetate-ethinyl estradiol-containing birth control pills (like that found in Diane and Diane-35) suppress sebum to a childhood range.[57]

Adults need more sebum than children, so your body reacts to this by ramping up its production of oil to create enough to keep your skin healthy. It essentially has to work harder to get over the threshold to make enough oil. After a few months or years of taking the pill, your body has become accustomed to making extra sebum.

Then, when you stop taking the pill, this increased oil production can persist for several months, but this time unopposed. This means that you have more sebum than ever before, and more acne and hair changes than ever before. This tends to peak around three to six months post-pill and then begin to subside. If you are in the first few months after coming off the pill and experiencing extreme symptoms – hang in there and know it will improve soon!

Another potential factor contributing to Post-Pill PCOS is HBC-induced insulin resistance. Several studies have shown that HBC can increase insulin production.[58] As you now know, excess insulin triggers our ovaries to produce extra testosterone, causing the main symptoms of PCOS. This usually begins whilst you are taking HBC and can persist for several months after you stop, similar to sebum production. As you wait for this to resolve, following the insulin resistance protocols in the next section can be helpful in improving your symptoms.

Finally, emerging research suggests that HBC has a mild antibiotic effect on your gut bacteria.[59] Alterations in healthy gut bacteria can trigger the onset of PCOS symptoms by influencing insulin sensitivity and androgen production.[60]

SPOTLIGHT: Janice's Post-Pill Journey

Janice joined one of my group programs after she had been on the pill since age 14. Her doctor had prescribed the pill to help her manage her mild teenage acne. It worked – her skin was clear and she didn't have to worry about getting pregnant before she was ready.

She had recently gotten married and at 29, decided it was time to start trying to get pregnant. Without giving it too much thought, Janice stopped taking the pill. She had one bleed when she first stopped, and then…nothing. Months went by and she had no signs of a period returning. To make matters worse, the acne from her teenage years came back with a vengeance! She visited her doctor who diagnosed her with PCOS and told her if her cycle still hadn't come back after six months, she would need fertility treatment.

Like so many other women, Janice had gone from spending most of her life terrified of falling pregnant, to being 110% ready to have a baby NOW. This desire was all-consuming and she came into the group program desperate for any advice to make her cycle return naturally.

I explained to Janice that it can take several months for your body to find "normal" again after being on the pill for so many years.

We put her on an androgen blocker to manage her acne and this cleared up within a few months. Meanwhile, we assessed her for nutrient deficiencies and corrected these. Janice had regular bloating and we discovered this was driven by low stomach acid, so we added some nutritional support to improve her digestion.

Right before the looming six-month mark, Janice had her first post-pill period. The very next month, Janice was pregnant naturally with a healthy baby boy.

Testing for Post-Pill PCOS

Unfortunately, there is no test that can conclusively confirm Post-Pill PCOS. This PCOS type is specifically related to when your symptoms started. If you're not sure if you had PCOS symptoms before you went on birth control, go back through the other three types, and take the quizzes to rate your likelihood of having these root causes instead of Post-Pill. If you are confident you have Post-Pill PCOS, you can skip ahead to chapter 15 for the core treatment for this PCOS type.

Signs of Post-Pill PCOS

- ☐ My symptoms started *after* I went off the pill (or another form of HBC like the Depo shot, an implant, or IUD) (**essential to meet Post-Pill PCOS criteria**)
- ☐ (Possibly) Elevated LH on blood tests
- ☐ (Possibly) High-normal prolactin on blood tests

There is only one essential checkbox in this section. If you aren't able to tick this box, you are dealing with a different root cause of PCOS. Read on to discover if Inflammatory PCOS is your root cause.

ACTION STEP:

Is Post-Pill your PCOS type? Tell us in the PCOS Repair Cysterhood Community and connect with other Type 3 Cysters! Go to nourishednaturalhealth.com/resources if you haven't already joined our free community.

Chapter 10

Inflammatory PCOS (Type 4)

The final root cause of PCOS is inflammation. All women with PCOS have some degree of chronic inflammation,[61] but in Inflammatory PCOS, this is the *primary* cause of your symptoms.

For this type of PCOS to be your *primary* root cause, you should have ruled out Insulin Resistance, Adrenal, and Post-Pill PCOS. This type of PCOS often overlaps with Insulin-Resistant PCOS because long-term insulin resistance causes inflammation and inflammation worsens insulin resistance.[62]

If you feel you fit the Insulin-Resistant PCOS picture covered earlier in this section as well as the signs of inflammation here, start by working on insulin before moving on to inflammation.

How does inflammation cause PCOS symptoms?

Inflammation is a normal part of your immune system response. We want inflammation in the right amounts because it is how our body sends immune cells to help us heal wounds and fight infections. For example, when you cut your finger, your body creates an inflammatory response to that area, bringing extra blood and immune cells to fight any bacteria that got into the wound and help close it up.

When inflammation continues for a long time unchecked however, this can lead to worsened PCOS symptoms. Chronic inflammation has been shown to stimulate your ovaries to produce higher amounts of testosterone.[62] This is similar to the way that high levels of insulin cause your ovaries to produce more testosterone. Higher levels of testosterone are converted into DHT, which gets into your follicles, causing acne, scalp hair loss, and facial hair growth. The testosterone affects your egg quality and causes issues with regular ovulation.

What causes chronic inflammation?

There are many factors that contribute to increased inflammation levels in your body. Autoimmune diseases, which involve the over-activation of your immune system, are a common contributor to Inflammatory PCOS. In these conditions, your immune system becomes disoriented. Instead of fighting foreign invaders it starts attacking your own tissues – creating high levels of inflammation.

Hashimoto's thyroiditis is the most common autoimmune condition I see alongside PCOS in my clients, and research shows that it is much more prevalent in women with PCOS.[63] Hashimoto's causes your body to attack your thyroid gland, creating damage that prevents your body from producing enough thyroid hormones, leading to weight gain, fertility problems, and fatigue.

There are more than 80 other autoimmune conditions, which vary in symptoms based on the body system they affect. All autoimmune conditions cause inflammation and tissue damage, which can contribute to the symptoms of PCOS by increasing testosterone production. Some of the other autoimmune conditions commonly occurring alongside PCOS include celiac disease, Psoriasis, and arthritis. Chronic skin conditions like eczema and hives also contribute to higher levels of inflammation through immune system activation.

Gastrointestinal disorders are another key contributor to body-wide inflammation. Conditions like irritable bowel syndrome (IBS) and small intestinal bacterial overgrowth (SIBO) cause a weakening of the lining of your digestive system, allowing particles of food to escape into your bloodstream. These particles float around in your blood where they shouldn't be, triggering your immune system to activate and start attacking them.

This is a common cause of food sensitivities and increased inflammation. If this is you, you might find that the list of foods you can't tolerate is growing by the day, or that you are often bloated or have alternating bowel patterns. Parasites, imbalances in gut bacteria, fungi overgrowth, and nutritional deficiencies are also contributing factors to increased inflammation.

Finally, a relatively common but overlooked cause of inflammation I have observed in women with PCOS is excess iron. Women of menstruating age are frequently low in iron due to monthly blood loss,[64] so iron excess is not commonly examined. In PCOS, however, long gaps between bleeds are a common feature. This means that if you have a genetic tendency toward higher iron levels, plus you aren't getting a regular period, you may be dealing with high iron levels. Iron is an important nutrient for energy and oxygen levels in the body, but in excess causes increased inflammation in the body.[65]

Signs and Symptoms of Inflammatory PCOS

Take the quiz below to rate the likelihood of inflammation being the root cause of your PCOS. Each time you answer yes, give yourself one point.

- ☐ I have ruled out Insulin Resistance, Adrenal, and Post-Pill PCOS
- ☐ I have chronic digestive issues like bloating, IBS, SIBO, constipation, diarrhea, reflux, or gas
- ☐ I have food sensitivities, allergies, or a chronic skin condition like eczema, rosacea, or hives
- ☐ I have an autoimmune condition like Hashimoto's, psoriasis, or celiac disease (or a family history of these conditions)
- ☐ I have been diagnosed with endometriosis
- ☐ My blood tests show low vitamin D levels
- ☐ My blood tests show high inflammatory markers (e.g., CRP), thyroid antibodies or gluten antibodies
- ☐ My blood tests show high iron or ferritin levels
- ☐ My blood tests show abnormal thyroid hormones or I have been diagnosed with hyper- or hypothyroidism
- ☐ I suffer from headaches, migraines, or unexplained fatigue
- ☐ I have chronic muscle or joint aches and pains or muscle weakness
- ☐ I am experiencing low moods or depression

If you said yes to four or more of the points above, there's a high chance chronic inflammation is the root cause of your PCOS symptoms, especially if you have ruled out the other three PCOS types. If you aren't sure or would like to confirm this with testing, see below for the best tests to confirm this. Testing is optional and if it's not within your budget right now, but you relate to the symptoms above, you can jump ahead and start implementing the Inflammatory PCOS Protocol in chapter 16.

Testing for Inflammatory PCOS

There are many causes of inflammation in Inflammatory PCOS, so asking your doctor to complete a range of tests to assess both your body-wide inflammation levels *plus* potential contributors to the inflammation is the best way to confirm this PCOS root cause. This way you'll be able to identify the most important areas to focus on to reduce inflammation (e.g., thyroid versus gut health).

<u>Tests to measure inflammation levels</u>:

- High sensitive C-reactive protein (hsCRP)
- Erythrocyte sedimentation rate (ESR).

<u>Tests to assess causes of inflammation</u>:

- Full thyroid panel (including TSH, T3, T4, and rT3)
- White blood cells
- Thyroid antibodies (thyroid peroxidase antibodies and antithyroglobulin antibodies)

- Gluten antibodies
- Vitamin D
- Iron studies (including ferritin).

ACTION STEP:

Is Inflammation your PCOS root cause? Tell us in the PCOS Repair Cysterhood Community and connect with other Type 4 Cysters! Go to nourishednaturalhealth.com/resources to join our free community.

Chapter 11

Still stuck? Is it really PCOS?

If you've gone through the four root causes in this section and still haven't identified a driver behind your PCOS, it might be time to explore if your PCOS diagnosis was correct. It's true PCOS if you have androgen excess as seen by either: *high androgens on blood tests* (testosterone, androstenedione, DHT, or DHEAS), *or significant physical signs of jawline acne, facial hair and/or thinning hair in the crown of your head.*[66]

If you have high androgens, all other causes of androgen excess must have also been ruled out to confirm PCOS.[67] Other causes for androgen excess include non-classical congenital adrenal hyperplasia, Cushing's disease, hyperprolactinemia, and androgen-secreting tumors.[67] These conditions are beyond the scope of this book, however your primary healthcare provider will be able to screen for these conditions if you are concerned.

> If you don't have excess androgens, you very likely don't meet the criteria for diagnosis of PCOS, even if you have polycystic ovaries or irregular or missing periods. Hyperandrogenism is the defining feature of PCOS.[68]

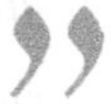

If missing or irregular periods is your main symptom, you might have been misdiagnosed with PCOS instead of hypothalamic amenorrhea (HA). HA can appear very similar to PCOS as it also causes missing periods and polycystic ovaries, however the root cause is very different. In PCOS, high androgens trigger your body to produce too much luteinizing hormone (LH), which shuts down ovulation, causing missing periods. As we covered earlier, these high androgens are either caused by insulin, cortisol, birth control, or inflammation.

In HA, the reverse happens. Undereating and/or over-exercising cause the body to deem your environment to be unsafe to reproduce. This triggers your brain to secrete *lower* amounts of LH, which also shuts down ovulation. Not ovulating regularly causes your follicles to stall in development, which explains why polycystic ovaries are often found on ultrasound in both PCOS and HA. If your PCOS was diagnosed by ultrasound alone, it's time to go back to the drawing board and determine if you truly fit the criteria for diagnosis.[66]

Treating HA is beyond the scope of this book, but essentially involves eating more calories, eating more carbohydrates, and reducing high intensity exercise. This allows your body to feel safe to begin ovulating again. As you can see, the treatment of HA is virtually opposite to that of PCOS. Instead of reducing starch to improve insulin, you likely need to increase starch and overall food intake.

Two of the best tests to confirm PCOS versus HA are follicle stimulating hormone (FSH) and LH. In PCOS, you will usually see a *high* LH to FSH ratio. In HA, you will usually see a *low* LH to FSH ratio. If your doctor isn't willing to perform further tests to confirm or rule out PCOS, it's time to find a new provider who can support you in uncovering what's going on with your hormones. Without knowing for sure that PCOS is the cause of your symptoms, the protocols in this book may not be appropriate for you.

STEP THREE: Heal Your PCOS Root Cause

Now that you have a clearer idea of what is driving your symptoms, it's time to develop an individualized protocol based on your PCOS type. Healing your root cause takes time and consistent effort, but once you do, your body will stop over-producing androgens. This means you will no longer need the androgen blocking principles we covered in the first section of this book.

Your skin will clear, your hair will stop falling out, your period will return on time, and those pesky facial hairs will no longer be an issue. You'll have the best, individualized advice for your hormones that you can continue to refer back to for the rest of your life.

I've covered the most impactful changes for each PCOS type in this section. If you are waiting on test results or aren't 100% sure which PCOS type you best fit into, follow the recommendations from the root cause that feels most likely or relevant for you. You will find many of the recommendations are similar between the four types, so you can get started with the basics and fine tune once you have more information about your unique root cause.

If you found you related to multiple root causes in the Identify Your Root Cause section, start with the one that you feel is most significant.

For example, many women fall into the Insulin Resistance and Adrenal PCOS categories. Eventually, you may need to work on both root causes, but to get started ask yourself: "Are sugar cravings and weight gain more of an issue for me right now (insulin) or is it my stress levels (adrenal)?". You will likely have an intuitive feel about the best place to start.

If you are really stuck, begin with the Insulin-Resistant PCOS Protocol as this is by far the most common root cause. Or jump into the PCOS Repair Cysterhood community and my team and I will help you work out which PCOS type is most likely for you.

Chapter 12

The PCOS Plate Method

Until now, you have been focusing on following the PCOS Repair Breakfast principles and eating your normal meals for the rest of the day. Once you are feeling confident with your breakfast changes, it's time to move on to lunch and dinner.

While we've kept your breakfast free of carbohydrates like starchy vegetables, grains, and fruit (except berries), enjoying some carbs in your lunch and dinner is really important. Contrary to what some social media influencers might have told you, women with PCOS *actually need to eat carbs* in order to ovulate.

Whether your goal is to get pregnant at some point in the future or not, ovulating regularly should be every Cysters goal because ovulation is the way we make progesterone. Progesterone keeps our skin clear, energy levels high, and weight stable, promotes sleep and relaxation, and protects against endometrial and breast cancer.

Not only that, but progesterone naturally inhibits 5-alpha reductase – the enzyme responsible for converting testosterone into its very potent cousin, DHT. Producing enough progesterone helps to grow hair on our head faster and thicker, reduces skin oil and acne, and stops unwanted hair growth.

The reason I never tell my clients to 100% remove carbs from their diet (even in severe insulin resistance) is because, as women, we have what's known as a "carbohydrate set point". This relates to a tiny part of our brain called the hypothalamus, which has an important role in constantly assessing our environment for signs of food shortage that would make reproducing dangerous.

Your hypothalamus looks for sufficient calorie intake overall, as well as carbohydrate intake specifically. Research suggests that every woman has a unique carbohydrate level that her brain determines as sufficient to ovulate.[69]

If you eat below this level of carbs for a long time, your brain perceives this as a lack of available food, and shuts down ovulation in order to prevent you from getting pregnant. While it might not feel like it, it's doing this to protect you because carrying a pregnancy to term requires an additional 75,000 calories – not ideal in a famine!

Both myself and my colleagues have observed that when women (particularly younger women) eat under a certain amount of carbs, even when there are sufficient calories from protein and fat such as in the ketogenic diet, they often lose their periods. There are very few studies in this area to date, however a 2003 study that put 45 people on a ketogenic diet for six months found that 45% of female participants lost their period or had irregular cycles.[70]

This phenomenon is not the same for men as they do not carry the same life-or-death decision to reproduce. This is why your male partner might have had incredible results following a ketogenic diet while you felt worse.

Because of this carbohydrate set point, I encourage you to keep your carbohydrate intake very low at breakfast time in order to promote stable blood sugar and insulin for the day, but to include a portion of gentle starch in your lunch and dinner meal.

By gentle starch, I mean starchy foods that don't cause inflammation in your body. All women with PCOS (regardless of your PCOS type) have increased body-wide inflammation in comparison to the general population, so sticking to anti-inflammatory foods is a great way to manage your symptoms.

Gentle starch sources include rice, oats, quinoa, buckwheat, and root vegetables (like sweet potato, white potato, pumpkin, squash, carrot). These types of carbs are not inflammatory. When paired with a protein source and healthy fat in a balanced meal, gentle carbs don't lead to insulin resistance.

Carbohydrates are important for sleep, which is why I encourage all PCOS types to include a moderate portion of gentle starch before bed. When you eat starch at night, it tops up your liver supply of glycogen (the storage form of carbohydrates) and helps to keep your blood sugar stable while you sleep. This is important for restful, restorative sleep and lowered stress levels.

Okay, so you're including some gentle carbs in your lunch and dinner meals to support your energy levels and ovulation, but how should you structure this? I created a simple method I call the PCOS Plate Method to help you adapt any meal to make it PCOS-friendly.

The PCOS Plate Method

When putting together a main meal, follow this simple hack to keep your macronutrients (carbs, fats, and proteins) in the right ratios to support hormone balance. Eating this way will support insulin sensitivity, keep stress hormones level, and lower inflammation – the three leading root causes of PCOS.

When you follow the ratios below, you will find that almost any meal can be made PCOS-friendly with just a few simple tweaks. See your PCOS-Friendly Food Formula bonus resource for ideas on foods to put in each category to build a meal. Ideally, opt for animal-based protein sources (like meat, fish, chicken, or eggs) as these contain high amounts of protein and minimal levels of carbohydrates.

Around one quarter of your plate should be made up of animal-based protein (this includes meat, fish, chicken, and eggs). Around one quarter should be starch – opt for "gentle carbs" to keep inflammation low. The last half of your plate should be made up of non-starchy vegetables. Finally, include a serve of healthy fat with your meal. You can drizzle this over your plate or use it to cook your protein or vegetables.

If you choose to eat plant-based proteins like lentils or chickpeas, remember that all plant proteins (except tofu) contain carbohydrates bound up with the protein. This means that legumes and beans fall somewhere in the middle of our protein and starch categories.

If you would like to include a plant-based protein in your meal, simply reduce your starch portion by around half, and up your non-starchy vegetables to fill the gap (see the diagrams below). For example, if you are eating a Mexican-style meal with beans, vegetables and guacamole, you will only need a small portion of rice or corn to go with your meal. If you had the same meal but with shredded chicken instead of beans, you could include a larger serve of rice or corn. If you are choosing tofu, follow the regular plate guidelines above as tofu contains mostly protein.

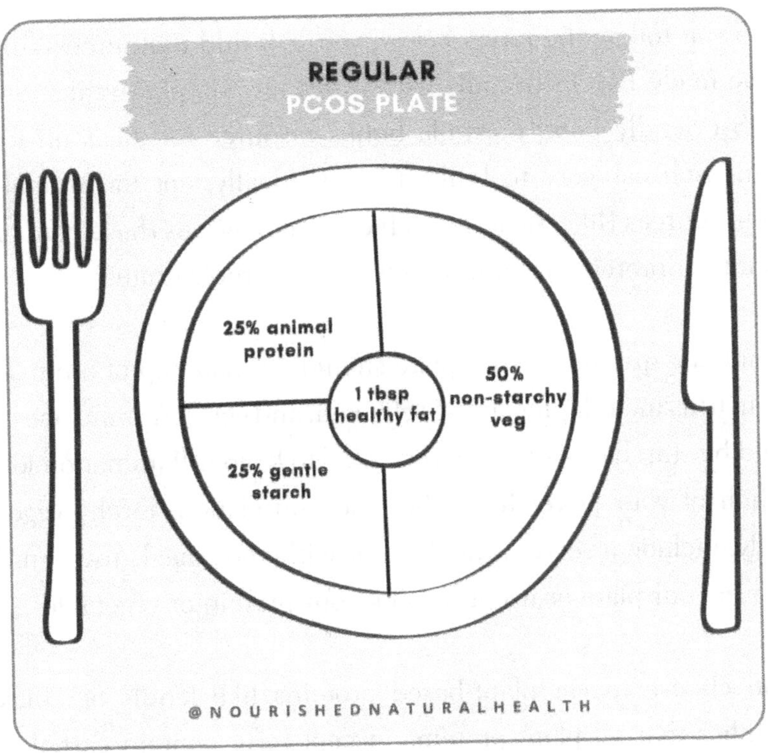

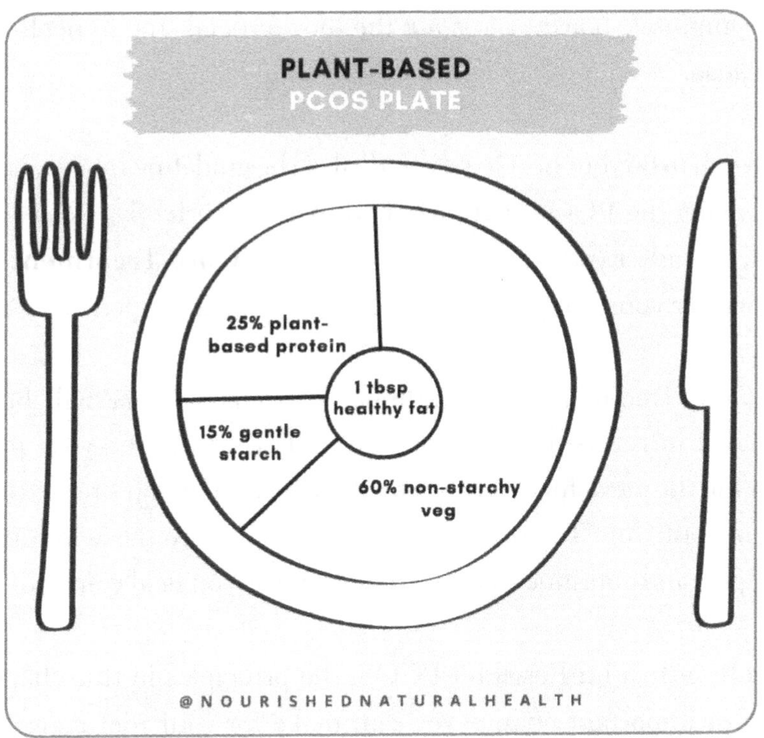

In your PCOS-Friendly Food Formula bonus resource, I've made following the PCOS Plate Method super simple. You'll find lists of foods for each plate category, plus some of my favorite PCOS-friendly meals.

Extra considerations for your root cause

Now that you know the PCOS Plate Method, let's cover some important tweaks to be mindful of based on your root cause. If you have identified Adrenal, Inflammatory, or Post-Pill as your PCOS type, following the PCOS Plate Method will be helpful in managing your symptoms, however it is *not* the most crucial step in healing your root cause.

I want you to do your best to be mindful of the guidelines above, however if following the PCOS Plate Method method perfectly is causing you stress, I'd rather you put your energy into the **Core Treatment** I have outlined for your unique root cause over the next chapters.

The Core Treatment is the number one change that will be most impactful in reversing your root cause. This should be your primary focus for the next few weeks. Once you feel like you are getting the hang of your Core Treatment, you can come back to these PCOS Plate principles and continue to implement them as you heal your root cause.

If you have Insulin-Resistant PCOS, the principles in this chapter *are* the most important change you can make for your root cause – *they are your Core Treatment.* Along with a few extra guidelines in the next chapter, the most impactful thing you can do for Insulin-Resistant PCOS is to work on what you are eating. Following the PCOS Repair Breakfast principles along with the PCOS Plate Method will dramatically improve your body's insulin sensitivity and begin reversing hair loss, acne, weight gain, and irregular cycles.

Can I eat fruit?

Whilst healthy, fruit contains fructose and glucose – two naturally occurring forms of sugar. Eaten in excess or alongside a large portion of starchy carbohydrates, fruit can cause a sharp rise in your blood sugar levels, which triggers excess insulin production, worsening insulin resistance.

If you have Adrenal, Inflammatory, or Post-Pill PCOS, enjoying any fruit in moderation should not be a problem for you, so long as you pair it with a healthy fat or protein source. For example, a snack of berries with coconut yogurt, a banana with some almond butter, or apple slices with peanut butter. You can also enjoy one serve of fruit alongside a meal like those outlined in the PCOS Plate Method above. The main meal will provide the protein and fat sources to blunt the rise in glucose.

If you have Insulin-Resistant PCOS, keeping carbohydrate and sugar levels lower is much more important for you. You can still eat fruit, but need to be mindful of balancing this with your starch intake. One serve of fruit can be swapped out for the starch portion of your meal.

For example, you might feel like having a piece of fruit for dessert after your lunch or dinner. To accommodate this, you could leave out the starch in your meal and up your non-starchy vegetables, and enjoy an apple or banana after your meal.

If you felt like a smaller portion of starch *plus* fruit for dessert, you could reduce your serve of each by half. For example, half a serve of rice with your main meal and half a banana for your dessert.

The exception to this rule is berries like raspberries, blackberries, and strawberries. These fruits are low in sugar and high in fiber, which means they can be enjoyed after a main meal without needing to reduce your starch component.

I never want you to cut anything out of your diet 100% because I know how this can lead to that familiar feeling of deprivation. Finding ways to still enjoy your favorite foods whilst balancing their ratios will be key in making this style of eating a long-term habit, not just another yoyo diet.

Chapter FAQs

I'm getting hungry after my meals following the PCOS Plate Method ratio. What should I do?

If you find you are getting hungry, try increasing your healthy fat source and opt for solid forms of fat like avocado, nuts, and seeds rather than oils. These are often more satiating because they take up more room in your stomach.

What about sugar, dairy, gluten, caffeine, and alcohol? Should I cut these out?

We'll cover whether removing or reducing these foods in your diet is an important focus for you based on your root cause in chapter 17. Cutting out foods can lead to feelings of deprivation and decrease the chances of you sticking with your changes. I only want you to focus on this if it will truly lead to big changes in your symptoms. For now, let's focus on the changes we've covered so far and, if necessary, we can add on another change when we come to it in the next section.

Root Cause Core Treatment

If you are confident in your PCOS root cause, feel free to skip ahead to the relevant section. Otherwise, if you are still confirming your type or are a combination, read through the Core Treatments for each root cause over the next few chapters to see which feels most relevant for you to implement first.

ACTION STEP:

How will you recreate your favorite meals to make them PCOS-friendly? Share with us in the PCOS Repair Cysterhood community and check out what other Cysters are cooking! Join us via nourishednaturalhealth.com/resources

Chapter 13

Insulin-Resistant PCOS Core Treatment

Changing what and when you eat, along with adding in some targeted nutritional supplements and finding joyful movement, is the Core Treatment for Insulin-Resistant PCOS. By now, you already know the principles to create insulin-friendly meals. Following these principles closely is a key focus to heal your insulin resistance and therefore reverse your PCOS symptoms. The Repair Breakfast Principles and PCOS Plate Method are Core Treatment #1 and Core Treatment #2 for Insulin-Resistant PCOS. See chapters 5 and 12 for reference if you've skipped ahead to this section.

Core Treatment #3: Reduce high-dose fructose

High amounts of a type of sugar called fructose can cause or worsen insulin resistance and abdominal weight gain. Reducing high-dose fructose in your diet is an important step in healing insulin resistance. High-dose fructose is found in table sugar (the kind that's used to bake cookies and cakes and added to your coffee and tea) and high-fructose corn syrup (the kind that you'll find in popular sodas). It is also found in some natural sweeteners that are often touted as being a "healthy alternative" like coconut sugar, agave, fruit juice, honey, dates, and dried fruit.

Fructose *is* present in whole fruit, however this doesn't contribute to insulin resistance because the amount is much lower than the processed sugars above. Whole fruit also contains fiber and other nutrients that negate the effects of fructose. This type of sugar is low-dose fructose and is not a concern.

SPOTLIGHT: How does high-dose fructose worsen insulin resistance?

When you eat an apple, the fructose present must be converted to glucose in your small intestine in order to be sent to your liver to be stored as energy. Low-dose fructose, like that in a single apple, isn't a problem and has actually been shown to *improve* insulin sensitivity when paired with regular exercise.[71]

High-dose fructose, like what you get when you eat a bliss ball or paleo dessert made with dates, contains so much fructose that your small intestine gets overwhelmed. All of the sugar isn't able to be broken down to glucose, and so it arrives at your liver and in your large intestine as fructose. This excess fructose contributes to fatty liver, oxidative stress, inflammation, and increased risk of insulin resistance.[72] It also affects your microbiome (the good gut bugs in your large intestine) and further contributes to insulin resistance.[73]

If you have Insulin-Resistant PCOS, *you don't need to stop eating fruit.* This is one of the biggest myths I see perpetuated in the PCOS community. While you are healing your insulin resistance, I don't encourage you to eat huge bowls of fruit salad, however a serve of fruit once or twice a day paired with protein or healthy fat is perfectly okay for PCOS and insulin resistance. Yes, you can eat bananas when you have PCOS!

Another common PCOS myth is that you need to cut out carbs while you are recovering from insulin resistance. When I first started healing my PCOS, I was literally *terrified* of potatoes. It sounds funny to me in hindsight, but at the time I felt lost about what I could and couldn't eat. I was so scared that carbs would make my PCOS worse that I would skip out on the rice or potato in my dinner, only to binge on a dessert made with "natural" sugars like agave syrup or dates. These "healthy" desserts were actually high in fructose, worsening my insulin resistance and PCOS symptoms.

Now I know that I am much better off having the carbs, feeling satiated and not needing a large dessert to "hit the spot." I include some gluten-free pasta, potato, or rice in my dinner and find all I need is a cup of peppermint tea and a square of 85% dark chocolate to feel completely satisfied. Not being controlled by sugar cravings after meals is incredibly freeing and I can't wait for you to enjoy this as well!

Instead of worrying about never eating a banana or potato again, I want you to focus on cutting all dessert foods and added sugars out of your diet for the next four weeks. I have found four weeks to be the ideal amount of time to reverse insulin resistance and get rid of cravings and reliance on sugar.

How to break up with sugar

If you feel like you are addicted to sugar – you aren't alone. Insulin resistance makes our brain *crave* more sugar and this can be incredibly hard to ignore. If you find yourself giving in to sugar cravings, I want you to know it's not because of your lack of willpower. It's because of your hormones.

Having suffered from severe sugar cravings myself, I know how all-consuming these feelings can be. What's important to remember is that strong cravings usually subside within 20-25 minutes, and after seven days of being sugar free, your cravings will likely disappear altogether.

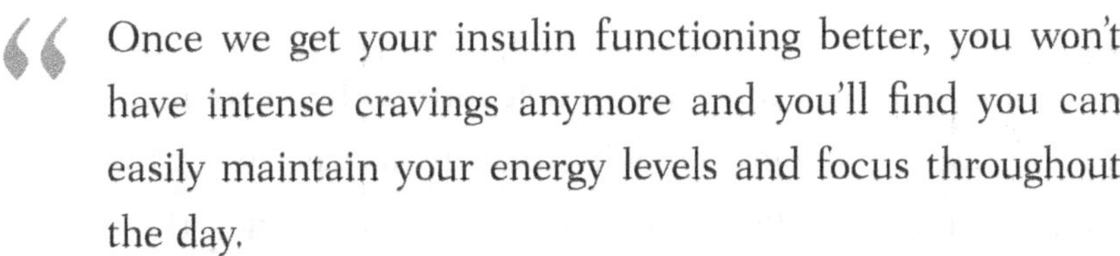

> Once we get your insulin functioning better, you won't have intense cravings anymore and you'll find you can easily maintain your energy levels and focus throughout the day.

For the next four weeks, your goal is to cut all sweet drinks (sodas, flavored milks, mixers), added sugar, and dessert foods out of your diet. *This isn't forever* – it's just for four weeks while we reset your blood sugar and insulin levels. This includes "natural" sugars like those in paleo desserts, bliss balls, and other treats that use dried fruit, agave, or coconut sugar. It also includes sweetened yogurt, granola bars, and protein bars.

You can still enjoy one or two serves of whole fruit paired with protein or healthy fat. If you need a sweetener while you are adjusting, try stevia or monk fruit as these are natural sweeteners that won't spike your blood sugar levels. You can also enjoy one to two squares of 85% or higher cacao chocolate as this is naturally very low in sugar.

While you are completing these four weeks, make sure you are having full, sustaining meals and snacks with plenty of protein. This will help to keep you feeling satisfied and reduce cravings for sugar. Remember that once we have reversed your insulin resistance, you won't have cravings for sugar anymore.

To help make quitting sugar easier, I've put together a bonus resource for you: Kick Your Sugar Cravings. There, I've covered many more tips to make this transition easier. You can find your free resource at nourishednaturalhealth.com/resources

After the four weeks are up, you can test your body's response to small amounts of sugar. I suggest enjoying one dessert or sweet food once or twice a week and really savoring the experience. Pick the day you are going to have a sweet treat and choose what you will make or buy. When you are ready to enjoy your sweet, sit without distractions and really be present while you eat it. Being mindful will reduce cravings for more sugar.

Once your insulin is functioning normally again, you can adopt the 80/20 rule we cover in chapter 22. This means enjoying a balanced, sugar-free diet 80% of the time, and choosing special occasions to enjoy small amounts of sugar or other foods that are less helpful for insulin.

Having insulin resistance now means you will always have a tendency to develop it again even after you have reversed it following the principles in this chapter. Finding a long-term, sustainable way to keep up these habits without feeling deprived is what will make all the difference to your symptoms.

Experiment with the 80/20 rule and find what works best for you. Ultimately, we want the PCOS Repair Protocol to form the habits you will follow for the rest of your life, instead of being another diet that you ditch for your old ways of eating after a few weeks because you felt unsatisfied or deprived.

Core Treatment #4: Choose your Meal Times

I am not a fan of intermittent fasting for PCOS, as outlined in chapter 5. Skipping breakfast can worsen PCOS by increasing cortisol and insulin levels. However, research shows that a gentle, 12-hour break between dinner and breakfast can be helpful for insulin resistance.[74]

This might look like dinner by 7pm and breakfast at 7am. Because you are ideally eating breakfast within an hour of waking to support your insulin levels, getting 12 hours between your dinner and breakfast might mean moving your dinner time meal a little earlier or cutting out after-dinner snacking.

This 12-hour window isn't a hard-and-fast rule – do your best, but don't let the timing cause undue stress. It will be more impactful to cut sugar for four weeks and focus on the balanced plate principles, so if this is all you can manage for now, start there.

Core Treatment #5: Consider Supplementing for Insulin Resistance

Along with changing your diet, adding one or two targeted nutritional supplements can greatly improve your body's sensitivity to insulin.

A blood sugar stabilizing supplement like PCOS Blood Sugar Balance can greatly improve your sensitivity to insulin, reduce sugar cravings and help you find a healthy weight. I designed this vitamin to complement the diet changes outlined above. The unique combination of cinnamon, magnesium, gymnema, and chromium has been shown to powerfully increase insulin sensitivity as well as reduce sugar cravings.[75]

Magnesium deficiency has been found to contribute to insulin resistance and supplementing daily has been proven to improve insulin resistance.[76] Chromium supplementation has demonstrated an ability to eliminate sugar and carbohydrate cravings, and reduce excess food intake leading to a healthy weight.[77] You'll find all of these ingredients in the PCOS Blood Sugar Balance supplement.

As well as this, you might like to consider an inositol supplement. As we covered earlier, inositol is a naturally occurring nutrient that has been shown to work more effectively than Metformin in sensitizing your cells to insulin, decreasing sugar cravings, restoring regular ovulation, and promoting weight loss. My top recommendation is Nourished Cycle Regulate + Ovulate as this contains the well-researched combination of myoinositol and D-chiro-inositol. You can purchase Cycle Regulate + Ovulate via nourishednaturalhealth.com/resources

Core Treatment #6: Find Joyful Movement

Moving your body is an important way of improving your muscle's sensitivity to insulin. Because of this, you might have been told that you need to do high intensity exercise to reverse your PCOS. Or other PCOS influencers might have told you that slow, weighted workouts are the only way to go. The truth is the research shows that *any* form of exercise is better than none.

My opinion is always: *the best exercise for PCOS is the one you'll actually do.*

Yes, there are forms of exercise that have been shown to improve insulin resistance more efficiently, but at the end of the day, I want you to find a style of movement that brings you joy. We'll cover the best types of exercise for PCOS in chapter 20, but for now, start experimenting with movement that feels good and where you're not watching the clock.

Remember that we are creating a plan that you can follow for the rest of your life, not just a few weeks. We need to find a form of exercise that you actually *look forward to* and can stick to in the long run. This could be walking with a friend, gardening, playing in the backyard with your kids, swimming in the ocean, or dancing to your favorite music. It doesn't have to be traditional "exercise," so long as it gets you sweating!

SPOTLIGHT: Shannon's Life Changing Journey

Shannon joined my group program after first receiving her PCOS diagnosis in her early thirties. As a teenager, she suffered from horrendously painful and heavy periods, which would last for two weeks and then disappear for four to six months at a time. She had excruciating cystic acne on her face, chest, back, and hairline and suffered the confidence-destroying effects of this for much of her life.

Her doctor prescribed the pill in her teens and she remained on this medication until she got married and decided it was time to start trying for a family in her early thirties. After many months and no positive pregnancy tests, Shannon visited her doctor and was finally diagnosed with PCOS. Her doctor told her she had two choices: to take fertility medication to get pregnant, or to go back on the pill because she was at risk of endometrial cancer due to her irregular periods.

Shannon knew there had to be a better way, so joined my program to learn how to reverse the root cause of her PCOS naturally. Over the next 12 months, Shannon's life completely changed. She improved her insulin resistance by following the protocols in the program. Her acne cleared. Her cycle regulated to a predictable 30 days. Her period became completely pain free. And she found a beautiful balance between following the Protocol and enjoying her favorite foods without guilt (more on the 80/20 rule in chapter 22).

Whilst on this journey to recover her health, Shannon also rediscovered herself. She turned her life around, separated from her husband, and found an incredible new partner. And at the time of writing this book, Shannon is blissfully pregnant with a healthy baby without the need for fertility interventions. You can watch Shannon's full story at nourishednaturalhealth.com/resources

Still having symptoms?

If you are following the Repair Breakfast Principles, PCOS Plate Method for lunch and dinner, meal timings, and low fructose guidelines but still experiencing symptoms of insulin resistance after several weeks – this section is for you. Try following the Repair Breakfast Principles for your lunch meal as well (i.e., low starch, high protein for breakfast and lunch). Make sure to still include a gentle starch portion in your dinner meal to top up your liver glycogen stores overnight. This will allow you to benefit from the effects of a low carbohydrate diet on insulin, whilst also ensuring you eat enough starch to ovulate, produce energy, and sleep well.

Summary: Core Treatments for Insulin-Resistant PCOS

- Enjoy a PCOS Repair Breakfast
- Follow the PCOS Plate Method for lunch and dinner
- Quit sugar for four weeks
- Try a gentle 12-hour fasting window

- Supplement a blood sugar balancing vitamin like Nourished PCOS Blood Sugar Balance
- Supplement an inositol vitamin like Nourished Cycle Regulate + Ovulate

ACTION STEP:

Which of these core treatments are you going to try first? Tell us in the PCOS Repair Cysterhood community. Go to nourishednaturalhealth.com/resources to join our free community.

Chapter 14

Adrenal PCOS Core Treatment

The *number one* thing I want you to focus on for Adrenal PCOS is balancing your cortisol production. When you are under stress, the same hormone which triggers your adrenal glands to secrete cortisol (ACTH), also triggers DHEA release. In Adrenal PCOS, adrenal androgens like DHEAS are the *primary cause of your symptoms.*

To balance your cortisol, we need to improve how you cope with stress, create a sustainable self care routine, and work on your sleep. These changes are more important for you right now than any of the diet changes we covered earlier in this book.

If you related to the Adrenal PCOS picture, there's a good chance you, like me, tend toward a 'Type A' or perfectionist personality type. This isn't inherently a bad thing – some of the most creative and high-achieving people have the same tendencies. However, when it comes to PCOS, this personality type can mean we commit 110% to areas of our life like improving our health. This all-or-nothing approach can make it hard to find sustainable ways to keep up with healthy habits without creating extra stress.

For all PCOS types, but particularly Adrenal PCOS, we need to find a balance between following a healthy lifestyle and pushing ourselves too hard. There is a happy medium that is possible to find with a little bit of experimentation. Scheduling in moments of downtime and relaxation will be just as important for you as making time for workouts or meal prepping.

You might find that your current exercise regimen isn't serving you or that there are tweaks you can make in your eating style to reduce stress. Or it might be your social engagements or work schedule that is causing you the most significant stress. Take an honest look at how you are living your life and which areas are causing you the most stress.

SPOTLIGHT: Hayley's story with Adrenal PCOS

Hayley* came to see me after struggling with her PCOS for three years. Like several other Adrenal PCOS Cysters, she did not suffer from irregular cycles. Her main symptoms were acne, hair thinning, and weight around her middle that wouldn't budge.

In an effort to improve her PCOS and ditch the weight, Hayley had joined a gym and was working with a personal trainer five mornings a week. Her trainer had her completing high intensity workouts for 45 minutes a day in the gym, plus long runs on the weekends. She was also strictly following a low carb eating plan as advised by her trainer. She ate the same breakfast, lunch, and dinner every day and felt very uneasy when she had to deviate from "the plan."

Hayley worked in a highly stressful environment as a secretary for a law firm and felt she was continuously "managing everyone else's expectations." When she came to see me, she was exhausted, stressed, and over it. She told me she couldn't work out any harder or eat any less, so she didn't know what to do.

We tweaked Hayley's exercise plan by swapping out three of her personal training sessions for a slow morning walk or yoga class. We also changed her diet plan to include *more* gentle starch like potato, oats, and rice as well as whole fruit for snacks. Hayley was terrified this would mean her weight would increase because she was eating more and working out less, but she agreed to stick with the plan for six months. I also got her to set her alarm ten minutes earlier to complete a morning breathing exercise that helps to lower cortisol levels.

After three months, Hayley's skin cleared and her hair stopped falling out. She felt energized, her brain fog lifted, and she felt she actually had the bandwidth to deal with the pressures of work. Her weight hadn't shifted, but she was feeling so much better in herself that she told me it didn't matter.

Then, around the six month mark, Hayley's weight suddenly dropped and she lost the extra weight around her belly. Hayley's story is a reminder that the calories in, calories out equation doesn't work when it comes to PCOS. Until you identify and heal your root cause, your body will not feel safe to shed the extra pounds. This is the same for insulin resistance and inflammation. When these body systems are out of balance, it is a warning signal to your body that you are in danger. Your body will try to keep you safe by dialing down your metabolism and holding onto extra weight as protection. When we can remove the barriers to healing by addressing your root cause, the weight loss will follow (with much less effort than you will be used to!).

**Name has been changed for privacy reasons*

Core Treatment #1: Empty Your Stress Bucket

Grab a pen and paper right now and write down all the things you can think of that are causing pressure in your life, whether good or bad. These can be tangible things, for example going to the gym, eating a healthy diet, catching up with your friends, or meeting deadlines at work. They might also be intangible things like expectations you have for yourself. For example, "putting pressure on myself to be the best mother/daughter/partner/sister I can be." Dig deep and try to get everything out onto the page.

When you have finished, take a look at everything on your list. Do some things stand out as more significant than others? Now ask yourself honestly – are there points on this list I could cut back on for a while for the sake of my hormones?

Some things on your list will not be possible to change, whereas others will be more movable. For example, could you make more time for relaxation on your weekends by saying "No" to one or two social engagements? I have a "maximum two events" rule for my weekends: Once I have said "Yes" to two things, no matter what else comes up, my answer is, "Thank you, but my weekend is already fully booked. Let's find another time."

Creating personal boundaries or non-negotiables is key to managing your stress levels and lowering your cortisol output. For many of us, releasing expectations on ourselves is another important aspect to reducing stress. If you know you have high standards for yourself in certain areas of your life, be honest and question if these are truly serving you. Could you let some of these expectations go and still feel fulfilled?

Core Treatment #2: Create a Stress-Lowering Morning Ritual

Now that you have made some more space for yourself in your week, it's time to create a morning ritual that will lower your stress hormones and set you up for a calmer day. How you start the day dramatically affects how you respond to unavoidable stress as the day unfolds. If you can commit to this practice, you will notice a huge difference in your overall stress levels within days.

Start by carving out around 10 to 15 minutes of time. I suggest scheduling this first thing in the morning, if possible. How you structure this is entirely up to you. The most important thing is to find practices that make you feel good and that you look forward to. Think of this as a beautiful gift to yourself that fills your tank before beginning your day.

Your ritual doesn't have to be a formal meditation practice. Below I've listed some of my favorite morning rituals to get you started. Pick two or three to begin with and experiment until you find a routine that works for you. You might like to mark your time by lighting a candle, burning incense, or playing some relaxing music (I love using a "Yoga and Meditation" playlist on Spotify).

Ideas for Morning Rituals:

- Five minutes of box belly breathing (in for four counts, hold for four, out for four, repeat)
- Coloring in
- Slowly drink a cup of calming, herbal tea (try spearmint for the bonus benefit of lowering androgens!)
- Light a candle, incense, or oil diffuser for the duration of the practice
- Journalling or setting intentions for the day
- Gratitude list
- Warm water with lemon (this also helps to prime your digestion)
- Gentle yoga or stretching
- Guided meditation (I like the free app "Insight Timer")
- Reading a relaxing (non-work or school-related) book
- Long, slow shower or bath

Core Treatment #3: Make Time For Joy

One of the quickest ways to combat excess stress hormones is to engage in activities that bring you joy. By joy, I mean activities purely for pleasure, rather than achieving things on your to-do list. When you are engaged in a joyful activity, the urgency of life tends to diminish a little.

So often as adults we forget to make time for the things we love in life because we are distracted by all the things we "should" be doing. The reality is, when you make time for joy, you will find you are significantly happier and more productive when you are undertaking the essential jobs.

Grab another piece of paper and write down all the things that you used to do that brought you joy. These might stretch all the way back to childhood. Write down as many things as you can, even if they feel silly or childish.

My client Emily really struggled with this exercise. As a mom of three, she told me she couldn't even remember what she used to do for fun before children. One day on the phone to her mother, she mentioned that Emily used to love coloring in as a child. Emily went out and bought an adult coloring book and now spends ten minutes a day coloring in after the kids are in bed. She told me she felt silly doing this at first, but now really looks forward to this moment of creative quiet at the end of a busy day. For her, it's the best way to stop, unwind, and lower her stress hormones.

Now that you have a list of joyful activities, pick one! Work out where you could schedule time for this activity into your week and make it a priority.

Core Treatment #4: Remove or Reduce Caffeine

In her book *Rushing Woman's Syndrome*, Dr Libby Weaver talks about the impact of the never-ending to-do list lifestyle on our caveman biology. Technology has increased at such a rate that things can be done faster than ever, but our bodies haven't caught up and we're feeling the effects.

In a desperate attempt to keep up with all of the pressures and obligations that life throws at us, we often turn to stimulants like caffeine to power us through. The problem with excess caffeine for Cysters with adrenal imbalances is that caffeine further increases cortisol and adrenaline production. As you know, more stress hormones means more DHEAS which means worsened PCOS symptoms.

While I know it's the last thing you want to hear, reducing or even cutting out caffeine for a few months could be really impactful for your PCOS. You don't have to do this cold turkey, and you likely won't have to do it forever, but for the sake of your hormones, consider how much caffeine you are consuming and if you could take a break from this.

Some Cysters are more sensitive than others to the effects of caffeine. You will know this because you won't be able to drink coffee after a certain time in the day, or you know you feel anxious after having some. If this is you, you are likely better off eliminating caffeine altogether for three to six months to allow your adrenal glands to heal. If you don't notice the effects of caffeine so significantly, you might get away with limiting your caffeine to one cup per day. (Note: this means *one* espresso shot or a small/regular sized cup of coffee, not a triple shot or a Grande!)

My top tip to reduce caffeine withdrawals is to go slow. If you usually drink three cups per day, drop down to two for a week and replace one with decaf coffee or green tea. After the first week, drop down to one weak caffeinated cup. Then, by the third week, replace all coffee with decaf or a single cup of green tea. If you feel good doing this, you could replace the green tea with decaf green tea to go fully caffeine free while your adrenals heal.

If you cut back significantly on your caffeine for a few months and don't notice any significant changes, you can experiment with adding a small amount back in and monitoring your symptoms. Every one of us metabolizes caffeine differently so finding your personal sweet spot takes a little experimentation.

Core treatment #5: Assess Your Exercise Levels

Are you over-exercising? Whilst regular exercise has been shown to lower stress hormones, overdoing it can have the opposite effect. You will know that you are doing too much if you still feel tired 15 minutes after finishing your workout.

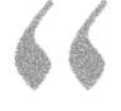

> Exercising should make you feel more energized soon afterward.

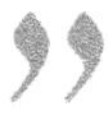

The 15 minute rule is a good gauge to rate how your adrenals coped with the exercise you just did. If you find yourself collapsing on the couch, this is a sign that your workout caused you to overproduce cortisol and adrenaline, which is not good news for Adrenal PCOS.

More than other PCOS types, we need to be mindful of the impact of high intensity exercise on our hormones.

I know how addictive keeping up a high exercise regime can be, but it's important to assess if your current routine is serving or hindering your results. If your stress hormones are particularly high, you may need to consider switching to slow, restorative exercises like walking, yoga, gentle pilates, or slow weighted workouts for the next few months while your hormones heal. You won't need to do this forever, just while you are reversing your root cause.

I've covered more specifics on exercise for your root cause in chapter 20, but for now, take a look at your current routine and be honest about where you could take a load off for a while so that exercise is energizing and stress relieving instead of exhausting.

Core Treatment #6: Balance Your Melatonin and Cortisol

Good quality sleep at roughly the same time each day is important for all PCOS types, but particularly Adrenal PCOS.

Our "sleepy" hormone melatonin naturally rises as the sun sets, helping us get ready for sleep overnight. In the early morning, as the sun rises, melatonin production drops off and is replaced by cortisol. Melatonin and cortisol are like two opposite ends of a seesaw. When one lowers the other rises to take its place. In a normal and healthy circadian rhythm, this rise and fall is balanced and follows the sun.

While we've covered a lot of the negative effects of too much cortisol elsewhere in this book, in the right levels, and at the right time of day, cortisol is important. It helps us feel alert and awake in the morning and gives us that "get up and go" feeling.

If you've been dealing with Adrenal PCOS for a while, there's a good chance your cortisol and melatonin levels are out of balance. You might find you drag yourself out of bed in the morning, need caffeine to get going, and don't feel like you are fully awake until lunchtime. Then right before you go to bed, you have a "second wind" and struggle to fall asleep. Your sleep is disturbed over night, so you wake feeling unrefreshed and the cycle continues.

One of the most important ways to improve your cortisol levels is to reset your melatonin and cortisol rhythm. We'll cover this in further in chapter 19, but for now, try these simple principles to improve your sleep-wake cycle:

- Try to go to bed and wake up at roughly the same time (even on weekends)
- Avoid screens one hour before bed (including TV) – if you need to use a device, use a blue light blocking filter like F.lux or blue light blocking glasses)
- Keep lights dim before bed – use lamps instead of overhead lights (or better yet – try candles!)
- If you struggle to fall asleep, try a short guided meditation before bed

- First thing in the morning, open the curtains and get as much light into your eyes as possible (without staring directly into the sun)

Core Treatment #7: Consider a Stress-Lowering Herbal Blend

Along with the principles we've covered in this chapter, adding one or two nutritional supplements to support your body's ability to cope with stress can dramatically improve and speed up your results with Adrenal PCOS.

My favorite herbal medicine for stress relief is ashwagandha root. This herb has been clinically proven to reduce chronic stress, lower cortisol, and lower anxiety.[78] Ashwagandha is an adaptogen, meaning that it helps your body adapt to stress. While the principles we've covered so far will go a long way in reducing stress in your life, some level of stress in the modern world is inevitable. My clients and I have found profound benefits from taking an ashwagandha blend like Nourished Calm + DeStress.

An eight-week study comparing ashwagandha root with a placebo found that perceived stress and anxiety scores significantly decreased in those participants taking the herbal medicine.[78] The participants taking ashwagandha also showed significant improvement in salivary cortisol and had greatly improved sleep quality compared with the placebo. Early research also suggests that ashwagandha may improve blood sugar control and diabetes,[79] making it the perfect Adrenal PCOS tool. Read more about Calm + DeStress at nourishednaturalhealth.com/resources

Core Treatment #8: Support Stable Blood Sugar

Keeping your blood sugar stable throughout the day is key to regulating cortisol levels. When your blood sugar drops too low (when you haven't eaten for a while or you ate a meal too high in simple carbohydrates or sugars), your body secretes cortisol. Low blood sugar is seen as a stress, and your body responds by releasing cortisol to help you fight (or in this case – go and find food before you starve).

We can prevent this feedback loop by making sure your blood sugar levels don't get dangerously low. To do this, follow the PCOS Plate Method from chapter 12. You might also find that you need snacks between your main meals so that you don't arrive at meal times ravenous. When snacking, choose a balanced snack that contains protein or healthy fat to prevent sharp rises and falls in blood sugar. For example: an apple with almond butter, a smoothie with protein powder, or vegetable sticks dipped in hummus and guacamole.

In your lunch and dinner meals, be sure to be including a gentle starch portion like we covered in chapter 12. Carbohydrates help to improve your cortisol output[80] and feed the healthy gut bacteria which produce GABA (the calming neurotransmitter we could all use more of!).[81]

SUMMARY: Core Treatments for Adrenal PCOS

- Empty your stress bucket
- Create a morning ritual that you look forward to
- Make time for joy (literally *schedule* it in your diary)

- Reduce or remove caffeine
- Assess your exercise levels
- Work on your sleep for cortisol and melatonin balance
- Supplement a stress-lowering herbal blend like Calm + DeStress
- Support your blood sugar with balanced meals and snacks

ACTION STEP:

Which of these core treatments are you going to try first? Tell us in the PCOS Repair Cysterhood community. Go to nourishednaturalhealth.com/resources to join our free community.

Chapter 15

Post-Pill PCOS Core Treatment

Hormonal birth control (HBC), like the pill, works by shutting down ovulation in order to prevent pregnancy. When you stop using HBC, most women find their cycles return within a few months without a fuss. For a smaller portion of women however, this suppression of ovulation *continues* for months or even years. Alongside this, a temporary surge in androgen production is common, particularly with brands of birth control pills that contain drospirenone or cyproterone like Yaz, Yasmin, Diane, and Brenda. This is why post-pill acne is a common symptom.

While your body finds balance again after being on the pill, it's common to be given a diagnosis of PCOS. Unlike the other three types of PCOS, this type is temporary. However, the symptoms can last for up to two years. In the meantime, following the core treatments below will help to reduce your symptoms and speed up your return to regular cycles.

Core Treatment #1: Stay Calm and Stick With It

For many women, one of the scariest parts about coming off birth control is the acne flare ups. If you've ever found yourself caught in the cycle of trying to come off the pill before, you'll relate to Ashely's story below.

SPOTLIGHT: Ashley's journey with post-pill acne

Ashley and I worked together after she had been on and off the pill four times in the past two years. She was ready to be free of medication and find a natural way to avoid pregnancy. Each time, she would boldly stop taking the pill and tell herself, "This is it – this time I'm sticking with it". Then three or four months later, her skin would be flaring up so badly that in sheer desperation for relief, she would end up back on the pill.

I explained to Ashley that post-pill acne flare ups usually peak around three to six months because of the unopposed sebum production and androgen surges from your ovaries (see chapter 9). This is why so many women give up hope and end up back on the pill at the three- to six-month mark. If you can wait it out just a little longer, things *will* improve.

Before quitting the pill again, we started Ashley on Nourished Androgen Blocker, removed some triggering foods from her diet like cow's dairy and processed sugar and worked on some underlying gut issues she had been dealing with. After two months on this protocol, Ashley felt confident to stop taking the pill once and for all, knowing she had a treatment plan in place. She had some mild symptoms in the first few months, but nothing she couldn't handle. She has now been free of HBC for more than 12 months and no longer qualifies for a PCOS diagnosis because her skin is clear and cycles are regular.

If you are currently taking HBC and planning to come off, I suggest implementing the core treatments in this chapter for around two months before stopping HBC. If you can do this, you will have a much easier withdrawal process with minimal symptoms.

If you have already come off HBC and are experiencing symptoms, *hang in there.* Follow the core treatment principles in this chapter, especially taking an anti-androgen supplement for quick symptom relief.

Core Treatment #2: Take An Anti Androgen Supplement

One of the major reasons we experience increased acne and hair changes after coming off the pill and other HBC is due to a temporary surge in androgens. The fastest, most effective way to stop these symptoms is to block your body's production of androgens. A herbal blend like Nourished Androgen Blocker is a great daily treatment to use while your body regulates its androgen production. Once your hormone levels go back to normal (usually around 12 to 24 months) you won't need this treatment anymore to control your symptoms.

Core Treatment #3: Avoid Cow's Dairy

Cow's dairy (but not sheep and goat) contains a protein called A1 casein, which in some women causes significant inflammation. This occurs even if you don't have gastrointestinal symptoms when you eat dairy (such as gas or diarrhea). Gut symptoms from dairy are more commonly related to the lactose content, rather than inflammation. A1 casein has been linked with several inflammatory conditions including acne.[82]

Unfortunately, there is no simple blood test to check if A1 casein is an issue for you. A common sign that you have an issue with A1 casein that I learned from Dr Lara Briden[38] is a history of recurrent upper respiratory infections during childhood. This includes chronic tonsillitis, ear infections, or bronchitis when you were younger. Researchers suspect that the inflammation associated with A1 casein contributes to immune conditions as well as acne.

Consider removing all cow dairy products (including yogurt, cheese, ice cream, and milk) from your diet for a minimum of three months to observe the difference. The exception to this rule is butter and ghee – the fat content in these products is so high that very little protein is present. You can also enjoy all sheep and goat milk products like cheese and yogurt, along with the many plant-based options now on the market like coconut, oat, and almond milks. Sheep and goat milk contain predominantly A2 protein, so will not cause the inflammatory acne effect.

If you are still taking HBC and preparing to come off, I suggest removing cow's dairy for two to three months *before* stopping the pill, and continuing for at least three months after coming off to minimize acne flare ups.

Core Treatment #3: Reduce High-Dose Fructose

Eating large amounts of a particular type of sugar called fructose has been shown to worsen acne.[83] High-dose fructose is found in table sugar (the kind that's used to bake cookies and cakes and added to your coffee and tea) and high-fructose corn syrup (the kind that you'll find in popular sodas). It is also found in some natural sweeteners that are often touted as being a "healthy alternative" like coconut sugar, agave, fruit juice, honey, dates, and dried fruit.

Fructose *is* present in whole fruit, however this doesn't contribute to acne because the amount is much lower than the processed sugars above. Whole fruit also contains fiber and other nutrients which negate the effects of fructose. This type of sugar is low-dose fructose and is not a concern.

I've covered fructose and how to lower your sugar intake in depth in the Core Treatment for Insulin Resistance in chapter 13, if you'd like to dive deeper into this. For post-HBC acne, I recommend reducing dessert foods to once per week while your skin heals. If you struggle with sugar cravings, check out your bonus resource: Kick Your Sugar Cravings.

Core Treatment #4: Replenish Depleted Nutrients

The oral contraceptive pill has been shown to deplete your body of essential nutrients including zinc, magnesium, B-vitamins, and selenium.[84] Zinc and magnesium in particular are crucial for regular ovulation and hormone balance.

Zinc is an ideal treatment for coming off HBC because it kills bacteria in your skin that leads to acne, reduces sebum production, lowers androgens, improves hirsutism (facial hair), and nourishes your ovarian follicles to promote regular periods.[85]

I designed Nourished Period + PMS Repair to replenish the vitamins and minerals lost whilst taking birth control. It includes vitamins B1, B3, B5, B6, and B12 along with a therapeutic dose of zinc and dong quai; a herb traditionally used to promote regular cycles and clear skin. Supplementing a high quality multivitamin that is designed to support female hormones like Period + PMS Repair for around six months is a great way to address the nutrient deficiencies that may be contributing to your Post-Pill PCOS symptoms.

Core Treatment #5: Support Your Gut Health

Research shows that the pill has a mild antibiotic effect on your gut microbiome.[59] We also know that 40% of women who take the pill have low stomach acid levels.[86] If you are dealing with gastrointestinal issues like bloating, alternating bowel patterns, heartburn, or indigestion, working on your gut health is important. Imbalanced gut bacteria can lead to gastrointestinal inflammation, further worsening acne and hormonal imbalances. Check out your bonus resource Beat The Bloat for my three-step protocol to healing gut issues.

Extra Considerations:

Do you have high prolactin on blood tests?

Prolactin causes androgen excess symptoms like acne and hirsutism by upregulating the 5-alpha-reductase enzyme – causing more testosterone to be converted to its super potent cousin, DHT.[87] If you have elevated prolactin and *normal LH* on blood tests after coming off the pill, the herbal medicine Vitex can powerfully reduce prolactin and promote regular periods.

Important note: You ***should not*** take vitex if you have raised LH. Vitex can cause LH production to increase, which worsens the symptoms of PCOS when used in the wrong situations. If you are unsure, speak to your practitioner for more advice.

If you have raised LH, the best treatment for you is a herbal medicine like dong quai that supports the regulation of LH and FSH. You can find a therapeutic dose of dong quai in Nourished Period + PMS Repair.

SUMMARY: Core Treatments for Post-Pill PCOS

- Stay calm and stick with it! Remember symptoms peak at three to six months and then subside
- Avoid cow's dairy (except butter and ghee)
- Reduce high-dose fructose (honey, dried fruit, table sugar)
- Replenish depleted nutrients – supplement a high quality multi like Period + PMS Repair
- Support gut health
- Check your prolactin

ACTION STEP:

Which of these core treatments are you going to try first? Tell us in the PCOS Repair Cysterhood community. Go to nourishednaturalhealth.com/resources to join our free community.

Chapter 16

Inflammatory PCOS Core Treatment

In this PCOS type, inflammation is the root cause of increased testosterone production in your ovaries. Inflammatory PCOS is the fourth category because it serves as a bit of a "catch all" for Cysters who don't fit into the insulin resistance, adrenal, or post-pill pictures. It includes many different "hidden" causes that in turn create inflammation and worsen PCOS symptoms.

To create your core treatment, we first need to work out *where* your excess inflammation is coming from. You could have an imbalance in your thyroid hormones, poor gut health, an overactive immune system, or be eating foods you are sensitive to. There is not one treatment for Inflammatory PCOS – it's a process of elimination to work out what will be most impactful for you.

You might already be confident in the most important areas to work on based on your symptoms or testing that you had done earlier to determine this PCOS type. If not, I've outlined some extra tests to consider to help you hone in on what's driving your inflammation.

Along with removing the source of increased inflammation, eating an anti-inflammatory diet and taking a natural anti-inflammatory supplement will help to lower your body-wide inflammation levels and support your immune system to be less reactive.

Core Treatment #1: Get your thyroid tested (everyone!)

The formal criteria for diagnosis of PCOS specifically mentions that hypothyroidism must be ruled out before officially diagnosing PCOS. This is because thyroid hormone imbalances can create similar symptoms to those of PCOS. Unfortunately, many of the women I have worked with have not had the appropriate blood work done and go on to discover their thyroid has been an underlying cause of their symptoms for some time.

Hypothyroidism (where your thyroid produces too little thyroid hormone) is the most common type of thyroid imbalance. Hypothyroidism causes increased androgen production and impaired ovulation – leading to irregular or missing periods and trouble falling pregnant. As you can see, these presenting signs are very similar to those of PCOS, and this is why diagnosis can often be missed.

It is also common to have *both* PCOS and a thyroid condition. Research shows that up to 25% of women with PCOS have thyroid hormone imbalances.[88] An underactive thyroid reduces your body's sensitivity to insulin, which contributes to the number one root cause of PCOS. Research shows that treating hypothyroidism improves insulin sensitivity.[89]

> If you have struggled to improve insulin resistance through diet and lifestyle alone, your thyroid might be what's holding you back.

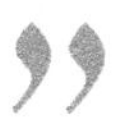

Signs and symptoms of hypothyroidism

- Weight gain (even on a low calorie diet)
- Feeling cold and low basal body temperatures
- Fatigue, feeling sluggish
- Hair loss
- Depression and low moods
- Dry skin
- Constipation
- Heavy periods
- Direct family member with thyroid disease.

Testing for hypothyroidism

If you have a di rect family member with thyroid disease, particularly if they are female (e.g., your mother or sister), there is at least a 43% chance that you will go on to develop thyroid problems yourself.[90] If you relate to the symptoms above or have a family history, visit your doctor for a checkup.

Hypothyroidism is diagnosed via a blood test. Your doctor might have told you your thyroid is normal based on your Thyroid Stimulating Hormone (TSH) results, however research shows that this test alone is not accurate enough to diagnose the early stages of hypothyroidism.[91]

The current guidelines state hypothyroidism cannot be diagnosed until your TSH is higher than 4.5 or 5mIU/L. However, many experts argue that this upper limit should be reduced to 2.5 or 3mIU/L.[92] Large population studies have demonstrated improved outcomes for pregnancy and fertility when TSH is below 2.5.[93] Ask your doctor for a full thyroid panel including TSH, T3, and T4.

Additionally, I recommend asking your doctor to check your blood for thyroid antibodies. Most cases of hypothyroidism are caused by an underlying immune problem where your body mistakenly attacks your thyroid gland, such as Hashimoto's thyroiditis.

In the early stages of autoimmune thyroid disease, raised antibodies are often the only sign. TSH tends to remain normal as the attack on your thyroid gland has not yet damaged the organ significantly enough to change your thyroid hormone production.

Ask your doctor to order thyroid peroxidase antibodies (TPO) and antithyroglobulin antibodies (TGAbs). The reference ranges for these tests vary in each country so follow the normal range from your laboratory.

If your doctor is reluctant to order these extra tests, mentioning the symptoms above which you relate to and/or that you have a direct family member with thyroid disease can be helpful. If you are really stuck, many countries have laboratories where you can request these tests privately (i.e., without the need for a referral). Please note these tests may not be covered by your insurance.

What to do if you have raised TSH and/or antibodies

Talk to your doctor or specialist about whether trialing a hormone replacement medication could be helpful for your PCOS. Prescription medications include T4 (such as thyroxine) or a combination of T4 plus T3 (such as desiccated thyroid). Combined with the lifestyle changes in the PCOS Repair Protocol, many of my clients have achieved incredible results by getting their thyroid functioning properly again. In some cases, this can be the final missing link preventing you from falling pregnant naturally.

Additionally, I strongly encourage you to consider removing gluten from your diet. A fascinating study found that people with Hashimoto's had significant improvements in symptoms and thyroid hormone levels when they removed gluten from their diet, regardless of if they had celiac disease or not.[94] Another study found that strictly removing gluten for one year single-handedly reversed thyroid abnormalities, whereas failing to adhere to the diet worsened the condition.[95]

Finally, consider taking the herbal medicine ashwagandha like that in Calm + DeStress. This herb has demonstrated an ability to regulate thyroid hormone production.[96]

Core Treatment #2: Heal Your Gut Lining

Research shows that women with PCOS have fewer healthy gut bacteria and more unhealthy bacteria than the general population.[97] This microbiome dysbiosis directly contributes to insulin resistance, weight gain and metabolic disorders.[98]

In a healthy gut, the cells lining your intestine are closely held together – keeping food inside. In PCOS, chronic inflammation causes damage to the gut lining, weakening the cells and allowing gaps to form. This is known as intestinal permeability.[99]

These gaps allow small particles of food and bacteria to escape the digestive tract and enter the bloodstream, triggering an immune response. This further contributes to inflammation, insulin resistance, higher levels of androgens, and problems with ovulation.

As you can see, inflammation both causes, and is worsened by, gut issues. If you suffer from regular bloating, indigestion, IBS, constipation, loose stools, or flatulence, improving your gut health will go a long way in reversing your root cause.

In my practice I have found the most common cause of chronic bloating is a condition called small intestinal bacterial overgrowth (SIBO). This is where normal bacteria from your lower bowel have migrated up to your small intestine where they don't belong. Bacteria in the small intestine ferment the foods you have eaten, leading to gas, bloating, and stool changes. The hallmark symptom of SIBO is painful bloating that lasts all day. Treating this overgrowth can greatly improve symptoms.

If you suspect you may have SIBO or your gut issues are severe, I suggest seeking out a practitioner who specializes in gut health. This person will be able to order the appropriate tests and assess your unique microbiome to provide you with an individualized treatment protocol. Like PCOS, the root cause of gut issues is extremely diverse and sometimes requires a deeper understanding that is beyond the scope of this book.

For general gut health maintenance, I have put together an extensive, three-step protocol: Beat the Bloat as a bonus resource for you. Access your copy at nourishednaturalhealth.com/resources

SPOTLIGHT: Rachel's journey with chronic gut health issues and Inflammatory PCOS

I first met Rachel when she had been living with severe gut issues for more than 10 years. She had long cycles (around 45 to 50 days) and acne which triggered her PCOS diagnosis at 19. She was chronically bloated, suffering from loose stools, IBS and a growing list of food intolerances.

In the past Rachel had tried Accutane for her acne which helped temporarily, but she found that her spots returned with a vengeance once she stopped using the medication. Rachel's gut issues were extreme, and we discovered that they were causing high levels of inflammation in her body, triggering her ovaries to make more testosterone. This extra testosterone was getting into her skin and causing acne, and making it harder for her body to ovulate.

It was clear that Rachel's gut issues were at the heart of her PCOS symptoms, so I encouraged her to work with a gut specialist alongside addressing her hormones. In severe cases like Rachel's, in depth stool testing can provide incredible insight into the unique factors that are triggering inflammation in your digestive system.

Through testing, we discovered that Rachel had very low levels of healthy bacteria, poor stomach acid and markers of chronic stress. She worked with her gut specialist to improve these markers. I helped Rachel find hormone-nourishing foods she could enjoy that wouldn't flare up her gut and we tweaked her high intensity exercise routine to include more restorative sessions. She found a new job which was more fulfilling and less stressful.

After two years of working together, Rachel had greatly improved her gut symptoms and her cycle reduced from 50 to 28 days. Her skin cleared and her most recent ultrasound revealed she no longer had polycystic ovaries.

Rachel's story is a reminder of the importance of finding the right team to support your overall health when improving your PCOS. By working with a gut specialist, she was able to make changes for her unique microbiome, and in doing so lower the inflammation which was driving her PCOS. For you this might mean seeking out an endocrinologist to help you with your thyroid, or a counselor to help you deal with stress.

Our body systems don't function in silos. When one area is out of balance, it has a flow on effect to other areas. Without working on the core issue of her gut imbalances, Rachel would not have been able to reduce her cycle length and clear her acne.

Core Treatment #3: Eat an Anti Inflammatory Diet

Minimizing foods that promote inflammation and filling your plate with anti-inflammatory foods is a great way to calm your immune system and lower your inflammation levels. Research shows that a diet rich in antioxidants and omega-3 fatty acids helps to lower chronic inflammation.

Along with the meal principles covered earlier in this book, aim to include foods from the list below to support your immune system and lower inflammation.

Anti-Inflammatory Foods to Eat More Of:

- Fatty fish like salmon, sardines and mackerel → these contain high levels of omega-3 fatty acids, which lower inflammation as well as support healthy hormone balance and stable moods
- Chia seeds and ground flax seeds → these are rich in ALA – a plant-based precursor to omega-3
- Olive oil → this has anti-inflammatory compounds like oleocanthal
- Dark red berries like strawberries, raspberries, blueberries, and blackberries → these are high in antioxidants that fight free radicals
- Dark leafy greens like kale, spinach, bok choy and silverbeet → these are packed full of many nutrients including vitamin K, calcium, and B-vitamins

- Nuts like almonds, walnuts, Brazil nuts, and seeds like pumpkin seeds and sunflower seeds → for their beneficial levels of vitamin E and selenium
- Cruciferous vegetables like broccoli, cauliflower, cabbage, and Brussels sprouts → which contain compounds that support detoxification of hormones
- Herbs and spices like ginger, turmeric, cinnamon, garlic, black pepper, and rosemary → these help to make food taste better and also contain anti-inflammatory compounds.

Start by filling your plate with the foods above. This will make it easier to "crowd out" some of the foods below that promote increased inflammation.

Foods To Limit on an Anti-Inflammatory Diet:

<u>Gluten:</u>

If you have an autoimmune condition like Hashimoto's, celiac disease, endometriosis, or rheumatoid arthritis, or if you have a chronic skin condition like eczema, I strongly suggest removing gluten from your diet completely for a minimum of three months and observing the difference. Research shows that gluten can exacerbate immune-related conditions, increase intestinal permeability, disrupt microbiome balance, and increase inflammation.[100]

If you don't have an immune condition but you are experiencing gut issues like bloating or IBS, consider significantly reducing your gluten intake for three months and slowly adding it back in to observe for symptoms. A condition called non-celiac gluten sensitivity (NCGS) is a common cause of a wide range of symptoms including bloating, IBS, stomach pain, headaches, migraines, foggy thinking, joint pain, fatigue, eczema, and mood disorders.[101] See chapter 17 for more information on NCGS.

If you have Inflammatory PCOS, the primary driver of your symptoms is chronic inflammation, therefore removing or reducing gluten is an important step in healing your root cause. This can feel overwhelming if you regularly eat bread, pasta, crackers, and other flour-based foods, but it doesn't have to be. There are so many great gluten-free alternatives out there that can be just as satisfying as the real deal.

Here are some anti-inflammatory and gluten-free starches to try:

- Quinoa (also packs a protein punch)
- Buckwheat (despite the name, this grain is gluten free and also high in protein)
- Brown rice
- All starchy root vegetables are gluten free (potatoes, pumpkin, sweet potato, beetroot, corn)
- Beans and legumes → these contain around a 50:50 mix of anti-inflammatory carbs and protein
- Oats → these are technically not 100% gluten free (unless marked as so) because they are usually processed in facilities that also handle gluten. If you have diagnosed celiac disease or a true wheat allergy, look for certified gluten-free oats. Otherwise, any oats are fine as the amount of gluten present is very minimal and won't impact inflammation.

Dairy:

Like gluten, cow's dairy can increase inflammation in some women. Cow's milk contains a protein called A1 protein, which can stimulate the immune system and lead to inflammation.

Sheep and goat milk products contain mostly A2 protein so don't cause the same issues when it comes to inflammation. This means you can most likely enjoy sheep and goat milk products without issues. You can also include ghee and butter made from cow milk as these products are mostly fat and contain very little protein.

Other great alternatives to cow milk are coconut milk and yogurt, almond milk, and cashew cheese. Oat milk is a common dairy substitute, however tends to contain fairly high levels of carbohydrates, so is best enjoyed in small amounts if you have any issues with insulin.

See chapter 17 for more information on dairy and PCOS.

Processed and Deep Fried Foods

These foods are not only low in nutrients but high in inflammatory compounds, which is not good news for Inflammatory PCOS. They also tend to be higher in sugar and refined carbohydrates that contribute to insulin resistance. Keep these foods to a minimum and focus on replacing them with the anti-inflammatory foods we covered earlier.

You'll notice many of these inflammatory foods are high in fat. We want adequate fat in our diet to support satiety and hormone balance, however opt for anti-inflammatory sources like avocado, olive oil, oily fish, and nuts and seeds instead of the processed forms below:

- Margarine
- Commercial cookies, cakes, pastries (and any other foods containing trans fat)
- Chocolate bars and candy bars
- Deep fried food including fries and battered food
- Processed meats: ham, salami, etc.
- Processed snack foods like potato chips
- Vegetable oil (like canola, soybean and sunflower oil) → olive oil, avocado oil, and ghee are best for cooking with

Core Treatment #4: Consider an Anti Inflammatory Supplement

Along with following an anti-inflammatory diet, consider adding a natural anti-inflammatory curcumin supplement such as Anti-Inflame + Mood. Curcumin is the active ingredient in turmeric and has been proven to lower body-wide inflammation in PCOS.[102] We combined curcumin with black pepper in Anti-Inflame + Mood to enhance absorption and directly support this root cause of PCOS. Find out more at nourishednaturalhealth.com/resources

Core Treatment #5: Correct Nutrient Deficiencies

Certain nutritional deficiencies and excesses can increase inflammation and cause your immune system to be activated, worsening the symptoms of Inflammatory PCOS.

It's worth assessing your current levels of vitamin D, vitamin B12, and iron through testing. If you find you are deficient, consider adding a supplement to correct this. In chapter 18, I've provided in-depth information about these nutrients, ideal reference ranges to look for on your blood tests and options for supplementing where necessary.

Less known but almost as common as iron deficiency in women with PCOS is iron excess (too much iron). This can directly cause inflammation and worsen insulin resistance.[103] Iron excess is particularly common in Cysters who aren't having regular periods as our monthly bleed is how we get rid of excess iron. If you discover you have high iron levels, consider donating blood to help lower your levels quickly. You'll not only be helping yourself but also your community! Ultimately, restoring ovulation and bleeding regularly will help to balance your iron levels.

Core Treatment #6: Reduce Exposure to Environmental Toxins

We know that exposure to environmental toxins while your mother was pregnant with you can predispose you to developing PCOS later in life. Emerging research is now finding a link between environmental toxin exposure and chronic inflammation. This topic can become a little overwhelming when you delve into it too deeply, however being mindful of some of the top sources of environmental toxins that you can easily avoid will be helpful in supporting your Inflammatory PCOS root cause.

One of the most common and most easily avoided sources of environmental toxins is plastics. We have known for a long time now that bisphenol-A (BPA) contributes to many health concerns, and research is now suggesting other plastics may have similar effects.[104]

The easiest way to minimize your exposure to plastics is to swap your water bottle for a stainless steel bottle and your food containers for glass containers.

Another common exposure to BPA is cash receipts. This is due to the ink used to print receipts. Ask for your receipt to be emailed to you, or minimize touching your receipts as much as possible. If you work in an industry that requires you to handle receipts, consider using gloves as a preventative measure.

The final environmental toxin to consider is pesticides. While avoiding pesticides altogether can be overwhelming and expensive, consider following the "Dirty Dozen and Clean Fifteen" list published by the Environmental Working Group.[105] This list outlines the most highly contaminated fruits and vegetables to prioritize buying organic, and others which are safer to enjoy non-organic.

Core Treatment #7: Find The Right Movement

The right level of exercise for your body can dramatically improve inflammation levels whilst also supporting your mood and healthy weight maintenance.[106] However, over-exercising can contribute to increased inflammation, so it's important to find your own unique sweet spot.

The best way to gauge if your level of movement is right for you is to assess how you feel afterward. You should feel energized and refreshed within 30 minutes of exercise. If you feel more fatigued, this is a sign that you might have overdone it. Similarly, some mild muscle soreness is normal after working out, but significant muscle or joint pain is a sign of increased inflammation.

Experiment with your current routine to find a balance that's best for you. While you are working on lowering inflammation, you may find that walking, swimming, or some low intensity resistance training is best for you. I've covered exercise for PCOS in depth in chapter 20.

SUMMARY: Core Treatments for Inflammatory PCOS

- Check your thyroid levels
- Heal your gut lining
- Eat an anti-inflammatory diet
- Consider an anti-inflammatory supplement like Anti-Inflame + Mood
- Correct nutritional deficiencies
- Reduce exposure to environmental toxins
- Find the right movement for your body

ACTION STEP:

Which of these core treatments are you going to try first? Tell us in the PCOS Repair Cysterhood community. Go to nourishednaturalhealth.com/resources to join our free community.

Chapter 17

Fine Tuning Your Core Treatment

Now that you have all of the most important changes in place for your root cause, it's time to fine tune your treatment for maximum results. You'll find the answers to many of the most common questions in this chapter like whether you need to give up gluten, dairy, caffeine, sugar, or alcohol. We'll also cover how to create PCOS-friendly snacks. Over the next few chapters, we'll look at nutrient deficiencies and testing options, the importance of sleep, the best types of exercise for your root cause, and how to get pregnant naturally with PCOS.

Do I need to go gluten free?

Celiac disease is an autoimmune condition where eating gluten (like that found in bread, pasta, and baked goods) causes your body to create antibodies that damage the walls of your intestines. This condition can be tested by measuring the presence of antibodies in your blood, as well as taking a biopsy of your intestine.

There is another condition however, called non-celiac gluten sensitivity (NCGS), which isn't as easy to diagnose as celiac disease as it isn't an autoimmune condition or an allergy.[107] NCGS causes a wide range of symptoms including gastrointestinal issues (bloating, IBS, and stomach pain), headaches, migraines, foggy thinking, joint pain, fatigue, eczema, and mood disorders.[101] Despite much debate, researchers have proven NCGS to be a genuine condition by giving self-diagnosed sufferers pills containing either gluten or a placebo. Those with gluten pills reported significantly increased symptoms that disappeared when they were switched to placebo.[101]

If you have Inflammatory PCOS, hypothyroidism, or an autoimmune condition, you will likely benefit from removing gluten from your diet for three months and observing the difference. If you can, visit your doctor to have your inflammatory markers and thyroid levels measured before and after the three months. If you notice your symptoms get better and/or your lab results improve, you will benefit from continuing to be gluten free.

What about dairy?

Like gluten, cow's dairy can increase inflammation in some women. It has also been linked with acne in several studies. Cow's milk contains two types of protein called A1 casein and A2 casein. Research suggests that A1 protein is likely the culprit as it reacts differently with your digestive system, stimulating your immune system to overreact.

Luckily, sheep and goat milk products contain mostly A2 protein so don't cause the same issues when it comes to inflammation and acne. If you have inflammatory PCOS, you can most likely enjoy sheep and goat milk products. You can also include ghee and butter made from cow milk as these products are mostly fat and contain very little protein.

If you have Adrenal or Post-Pill PCOS, sheep and goat milk products are a great choice, as are hard cheeses made from cow milk (like cheddar and parmesan). If acne or digestive issues are not major symptoms, small amounts of yogurt is likely okay for you as well.

If you have Insulin-Resistant PCOS, you need to be a little stricter with all dairy to keep your insulin levels low. Dairy contains growth hormones like insulin-like growth factor 1 (IGF-1) and branched-chain amino acids (BCAAs). These hormones are powerful growth hormones that are designed to grow a baby calf into a large cow. In humans, they cause a spike in insulin production.

Low fat dairy in particular is one of the most insulin-stimulating foods (more so than white bread!). Because of this, if you have insulin resistance, I suggest avoiding all forms of dairy except for butter and ghee. If you are really craving some cheese as a treat, go for a small amount of hard cheese as this will have less impact on your insulin.

If acne is one of your major symptoms, regardless of your PCOS type, consider following the Insulin Resistance advice above. IGF-1 and BCAAs stimulate insulin production, which increases testosterone from your ovaries, and in turn that upregulates oil production in your skin, causing blocked pores and acne.

If you are struggling to reduce dairy, there are many delicious non-dairy products available that taste very similar to the real deal. I love almond milk in my morning smoothie and coconut yogurt with fruit as a snack. When choosing non-dairy products, read the label and check for added sugars and other ingredients that may not be PCOS-friendly. Be mindful of other places you might be including dairy such as your protein powder or protein bars. Swap whey protein for pea, collagen, brown rice, or egg white protein to support healthy insulin levels and clear skin.

Do I need to give up coffee?

If you have Adrenal PCOS, you already know that reducing or removing caffeine entirely is an important part of healing your excess cortisol and DHEAS production. If you don't have Adrenal PCOS, there is a little more flexibility.

In my practice, I have observed that all PCOS types benefit from a reduction in caffeine due to the lowering of cortisol. However, what's more important for all other PCOS types are the core treatments outlined earlier in the book.

For now, I suggest you focus on implementing the core treatments unless you know you are particularly sensitive to caffeine or that you feel much more anxious and stressed when you drink it. Several months from now, once you are confidently following your Root Cause Core Treatment and are noticing improvements, you might consider reducing or removing caffeine and observing the difference.

Should I skip dessert?

If you have Insulin-Resistant PCOS, you already know that removing added sugar and high-dose fructose for four weeks is an integral part of healing your insulin resistance. Avoiding dessert foods and sweeteners is more important for insulin resistance than avoiding gentle starch like bread, potatoes, and pasta.

If you have Adrenal, Post-Pill, or Inflammatory PCOS, you can likely get away with some small serves of dessert once or twice a week. Coupled with regular exercise, research shows that including small amounts of sugar in your diet has minimal impact.[71] If you aren't exercising or have insulin resistance, you are best avoiding added sugar and "natural" sweeteners like dates, agave syrup and coconut sugar. This includes protein balls made with dates and other dried fruit.

If you do choose to include some dessert foods in your diet, follow the 80/20 rule (see chapter 22). Pick a food or flavor you are really craving, make time to enjoy it and really savor the experience. Some of my favorite PCOS-friendly desserts include frozen berries and frozen bananas blended with coconut cream (to create an ice cream consistency) and dark chocolate with peanut butter.

Alcohol and PCOS – no more Friday night wines?

Unlike some of the other foods and drinks in this chapter, it will be no surprise to you that excess alcohol consumption is not good for health. Alcohol increases inflammation, contributes to your sugar intake, disturbs sleep, and can affect fertility and gut health. If you are currently trying to conceive, I strongly suggest removing alcohol entirely as alcohol consumption is a risk factor for miscariage and poor egg quality.[108] Research also suggests that your partner's alcohol intake can affect sperm quality, so consider getting your partner on board as well.

If you aren't currently trying to conceive, I suggest limiting alcohol to a maximum of two to three drinks per week. Avoid drinking on an empty stomach and aim to enjoy alongside a main meal if possible. Be mindful of added sugar in drinks such as mixers as these can quickly spike glucose and insulin levels.

Finally, if you take Metformin for your PCOS, alcohol intake is advised against as this medication increases your risk of lactic acidosis, which is increased with alcohol consumption.

Can I snack when I have PCOS?

We've covered breakfast, lunch, and dinner in depth in earlier chapters in the PCOS Repair Protocol. If you are following these guidelines, you might find that you don't feel the need to snack anymore as your hunger and fullness cues become more balanced. If you are genuinely hungry between meals or find you are ravenous by main meal time, please choose a balanced snack to keep your blood sugar levels stable.

The principles for creating PCOS-friendly snacks are similar to those we covered for your main meals. Always include a protein or healthy fat source (or both), and avoid "naked" carbohydrates, for example, a piece of fruit or a cracker on its own.

Eating an apple causes a quick rise in blood sugar levels, which triggers insulin to be secreted to bring it back down. If you were to take that same apple and eat it alongside a handful of nuts or some coconut yogurt, the fat and protein would help to blunt the rise in glucose because fat and protein are absorbed more slowly. This means your body doesn't need to release as much insulin.

Eating snacks following this method will keep your insulin levels low and will sustain you for longer until your next main meal.

Some of my favorite PCOS-friendly snacks include:

- Fresh berries and coconut yogurt
- Apple with almond butter
- ½ fresh capsicum (bell pepper) filled with mashed avocado or hummus
- Hard boiled egg
- Seed crackers with hummus or goat cheese (if tolerated)
- Homemade protein balls with nut butter, protein powder, and almond meal
- Handful of mixed nuts
- Small tin of tuna or salmon with seed crackers

ACTION STEP:

Check out the PCOS Repair Cysterhood community for more snack suggestions from other Cysters! Make sure to share your favorite recipes with us as well. Go to nourishednaturalhealth.com/resources to join our free community.

Chapter 18

Nutrient Deficiencies, Testing, and Supplements

Over the years, I have observed several common nutrient deficiencies in women with PCOS. These deficiencies can increase inflammation, make us feel tired, impede ovulation, and worsen insulin resistance. Sometimes, a nutrient deficiency can be a "hidden cause" preventing you from healing your PCOS. The following tests are worth requesting for a full overview of the contributing factors to your symptoms as well as your root cause.

Vitamin D

One of the most important nutrients for PCOS is vitamin D. Many people around the world don't get enough sunshine to produce adequate amounts of vitamin D through their skin. Studies show that 67-85% of women with PCOS are deficient in vitamin D.[109] High cortisol levels (such as those in Adrenal PCOS) have also been shown to deplete vitamin D levels.

Vitamin D functions as a hormone and deficiency has been shown to exacerbate insulin resistance, irregular cycles, fertility problems, hirsutism, hyperandrogenism, and obesity.[110] Research suggests that vitamin D plays an integral role in insulin secretion and sensitivity and that low levels are correlated with type 2 diabetes.[111]

Improving vitamin D status has been associated with higher chances of falling pregnant and carrying a baby to term in women with PCOS who have fertility issues.[112] Beyond hormones, vitamin D is also a crucial nutrient for your immune system and deficiency can increase inflammation and immune reactivity. Sufficient levels are important for *all* root causes of PCOS.

The best way to assess your vitamin D status is through a blood test. It's a good idea to have this tested roughly every six months to assess the impact of different seasons and supplementation on your blood levels. An ideal blood vitamin D level is between 87-150nmol/L (27-47ng/dL).

The easiest way to improve vitamin D levels is through a supplement. The research for PCOS shows that we likely need around 2000-4000 IU of vitamin D daily just to maintain our normal levels if we aren't getting adequate sunlight. If through testing you find you are deficient, you will likely need a dose of at least 4000 IU for a few months to replenish your levels. Talk to your doctor about what level of supplementation would be most appropriate for you.

Vitamin B12

B12 is a crucial nutrient for energy production, brain function, and many other processes in the body. B12 deficiency is common in women with PCOS due to poor absorption and/or poor intake. It is found almost exclusively in animal based foods, so vegetarian and vegan women are at a higher risk of B12 deficiency. Also, Metformin has been shown to deplete vitamin B12 levels, so this is even more important to assess if you have a history of Metformin use.

B12 levels can be measured through a simple blood test. Ideal ranges are 332-1475pmol/L (90-401pg/mL). A simple daily supplement can increase suboptimal levels. If you find you are severely deficient, talk to your doctor about the pros and cons of a B12 injection to quickly boost your levels.

Iron

You have likely heard of the importance of adequate iron levels for menstruating women. It's common for women to be low in iron, leading to fatigue, brain fog, and other issues. Because of this, it's common for women of reproductive age to be taking an iron supplement.

Interestingly, I have observed a tendency for iron excess (too much iron) almost as frequently as low iron in my PCOS clients. Iron excess has been shown to significantly increase inflammation and worsen insulin resistance.[103] This is more common in Cysters who aren't having regular periods, as this is our main way of getting rid of extra iron each month.

Before taking an iron supplement, it's really important to check your blood levels to make sure you are truly deficient. There are four blood tests to check your iron status and these can be requested from your doctor as a "full iron panel." They include:

- Ferritin – this shows how much iron you have stored
- Transferrin saturation – helps us see if you store too much iron
- Total iron – shows us how much is present in your blood
- Hemoglobin – will be low if you have a condition called iron deficiency anemia.

Ferritin is the most important of these four tests. Ideally, you should have a range between 30-100 micromole per liter (μmol/L). If your levels are too low, consider a supplement containing iron bisglycinate as this is less likely to cause constipation like other forms of iron. If your levels are too high, consider donating blood as a way to lower your levels as well as working on getting regular periods again.

Magnesium

This important mineral is involved in over 300 reactions in the body. It plays an important role in reducing inflammation so is a great treatment for Inflammatory PCOS. It is also involved in glycemic control and researchers have found links between low magnesium and insulin resistance.[113]

Unfortunately, there is no accurate way to measure your magnesium levels, as we store most of our magnesium in our tissues and bones, not in our blood. However, research shows that around 20% of the general population are magnesium deficient[114] and 75% of people with type 2 diabetes have low levels.[115] This means there is a reasonable chance that your levels are suboptimal.

Magnesium supplementation at standard dosages is generally regarded as safe as it doesn't cause a build up in your body like too much iron. It also has the added benefit of reducing sugar cravings, improving energy levels, and promoting regular ovulation. I recommend magnesium glycinate or magnesium bisglycinate as these are the most well absorbed forms of magnesium that won't cause digestive issues. A standard dose of magnesium is around 300-400mg per day.

Chapter 19

Sleep for Cysters

Having PCOS means you need more consistent sleep to feel energized than your non-PCOS friends. To make things more difficult, it's often harder to sleep well when you have PCOS. The hormonal dysregulation of PCOS can impact on your circadian rhythm, making it harder to fall asleep at the right time and feel refreshed the next morning. On top of this, sleep apnoea (a sleep breathing disorder) is frequently associated with PCOS. This is why fatigue is such a common symptom for many Cysters.

Not getting enough sleep impacts *all* root causes of PCOS. It reduces your cells' sensitivity to insulin, increases cortisol output, and contributes to inflammation. Just one night of poor sleep has been shown to increase insulin resistance.[49] As well as this, sleep deprivation makes us crave sugar and other refined carbohydrates for a quick energy boost.

These simple forms of carbohydrates are easily broken down into energy so quickly raise our blood sugar levels, but they also raise our insulin, further contributing to insulin resistance.

> "Being tired makes it harder for us to make good decisions and exercise our willpower, so it's no wonder we find it harder to say "No" to chocolate and pastries after a restless night!

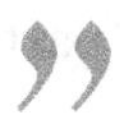

Not sleeping enough also increases chronic inflammation. A recent study found that seven nights of reduced sleep significantly increased inflammatory biomarkers, particularly in women.[116] Finally, sleep deprivation is a form of stress on our body and increases cortisol production, contributing to Adrenal PCOS.

Six Tips to Improve Sleep

1. Sleep in total darkness

Our brain relies on the cue of darkness to produce melatonin (our sleepy hormone) and balance our circadian rhythm. Light in the bedroom, particularly blue light, can trick our brain into thinking it's still daytime, and reduce its melatonin output. Turn the lights out in your bedroom at night and assess any sources of light that you can reduce. For example, bright street lights that you could block with thicker curtains, a radio clock, or other electronic light.

If you can't make your room dark enough to not be able to see your hand in front of your face, consider buying an eye mask to easily create total darkness.

2. Sleep in quiet and cool

Many of us don't realize the impact of noise on our sleep. Snoring partner? Noisy street traffic? If there are noises you can't change in your sleep environment, consider buying a pair of earplugs or using a white noise machine.

In order to fall asleep, our core body temperature must drop slightly. Make sure you are using the appropriate thickness blanket on your bed and have a fan or air conditioner for warmer nights.

3. Find a routine

Our bodies rely on cues for when it's time to wind down. Find a bedtime routine that you enjoy and that serves as a signal to your brain to start producing melatonin. It might involve taking a bath, reading a book, drinking herbal tea, or doing a short meditation. Avoid screens at much as possible in the hour before bedtime as these contribute to the blue light mentioned above. If you absolutely need to work on your computer or use your phone, use a blue light blocker like "F.lux" on your computer, "Night Shift" on your iPhone, or a bedtime app on other devices.

4. Stay out of bed (except for sleep!)

Our brains love associations, so keep your bed for sleeping only (apart from sex!). Avoid watching TV, checking emails, or spending time on your phone in bed. This will help to reduce racing thoughts while you are trying to sleep.

If you do find yourself thinking or trying to remember things while you are sleeping, try keeping a notepad and pen on your bedside table. That way, you can jot down anything that's on your mind and then let it go instead of letting it keep you awake.

5. Mind still racing? Try a five to ten minute meditation

If you know you have a very active brain the minute the lights go out, try a short guided meditation to help you relax before bed. This will help you leave the to-do lists behind and drop into the present moment.

6. Cut the coffee

If you are drinking coffee after lunchtime, consider swapping this for herbal tea as the caffeine may be disrupting your circadian rhythm.

Still stuck?

You might benefit from a melatonin supplement. This will naturally support your body's own melatonin production and help to establish your circadian rhythm. Melatonin is particularly helpful if you feel "tired but wired" when going to bed at night, take longer than 15 to 20 minutes to fall asleep or wake frequently during the night.

Along with improving sleep, melatonin supplementation has been studied for its metabolic and hormonal effects in women with PCOS. Interestingly, our ovaries have receptors for melatonin and require sufficient levels to function optimally. Women with PCOS are more likely to have low melatonin levels, and it is theorized that this may contribute to some of the hallmark symptoms of PCOS.

One study found that melatonin supplementation reduced androgen and insulin levels.[117] A large review found that melatonin supplementation enhanced egg quality, reduced obesity, and lowered inflammation in PCOS.[118]

If you would like to try supplementing, start with 1mg around 30 minutes before bed and slowly increase your dose each night until you find the right amount for your body. You should feel sleepy and relaxed within 20 minutes of taking the melatonin, but not wake up feeling groggy the next morning.

ACTION STEP:

Do you struggle to get enough sleep? Which of these six steps are you going to try to improve your sleep? Tell us in the PCOS Repair Cysterhood community what you're doing for more shut-eye. Go to nourishednaturalhealth.com/resources to join our free community.

Chapter 20

Movement and Exercise for PCOS

When it comes to movement and PCOS, finding the right balance is key. Both too much and too little exercise can worsen PCOS symptoms. In this chapter, we'll cover how to work out if you are over or under exercising as well as the best form of exercise for PCOS.

Are you overdoing exercise?

Over exercising can be harmful for all root causes of PCOS. An interesting study found that moderately-high to high intensity exercise (such as a spin or HIIT class) increased cortisol levels, whereas low intensity exercise lowered cortisol.[119] Higher cortisol levels trigger your adrenal glands to release excess DHEAS which in turn increase the symptoms of PCOS like acne, hair changes, and irregular cycles.

What's more, the study found that this increased cortisol production persisted for several hours after completing the workout. For the 80% of Cysters with Insulin-Resistant PCOS, this is an issue because high cortisol levels trigger your body to release glucose into your bloodstream.

If, like many of us, you spend the majority of your day sitting at a desk, this extra glucose isn't used by your muscles. Having too much glucose sitting in your blood is dangerous, so your body increases its production of insulin to bring the levels down. Over time, this can worsen insulin resistance as well as increase inflammation.

So how do you know if you are overdoing exercise? Look at how quickly you recover after finishing a workout or session. You should recover and feel more energized within 30 minutes. If you feel more fatigued, this is a sign that you overdid it. When one of my clients, Sammi, first came to see me she proudly announced that she worked out so intensely that she would collapse on the couch or need to take a nap afterward. Exercising to fatigue is not a sign of a "good" workout and is not sustainable.

The other telltale sign is changes to your sleep. If you notice you take longer than 20 minutes to fall asleep at night, wake frequently throughout the night, or wake up feeling unrefreshed even after enough hours in bed, this is a sign that your stress hormones may be out of whack. Try reducing the intensity of your exercise for a few days whilst keeping your other habits similar to observe if your workouts might be impacting your sleep.

Are you getting *enough* exercise?

Getting some form of movement into your week is important for improving insulin resistance, lowering inflammation, and keeping stress hormones at bay. The International Evidence Based Guidelines for PCOS recommend "a minimum of 150 min/week of moderate intensity physical activity or 75 min/week of vigorous intensities or an equivalent combination of both, including muscle strengthening activities on 2 non-consecutive days/week".[120] This could be a 15-minute walk to and from your car or the train station each work day, plus some simple squats and lunges twice a week at home. If exercise is new for you, start small and build from there.

The "best" exercise for PCOS

Despite what you might have heard from influencers, there is no one "perfect" exercise for PCOS. The best exercise plan for you is the one you actually enjoy and will keep on doing. Remember that to control your PCOS symptoms, you will need to follow the PCOS Repair principles for the rest of your life, not just a few weeks. We are creating sustainable habits that you can stick with, instead of just another fad you can't sustain. Taking the time to experiment with different forms of movement is important in determining what works for you.

If you are open to different types of exercise and would like to maximize your results, I have found my clients have great results with a combination of HIIT or strength-based exercises plus low intensity movement. This might look like two or three 20-minute HIIT/bodyweight sessions per week, plus a 30-minute walk or cycle most days. It might be more or less than this based on your root cause, your current fitness level, and your schedule. For Adrenal PCOS with very high stress levels, you might like to skip HIIT sessions for now, or keep them to under ten minutes while your stress hormones recover.

HIIT exercise involves short bursts of high intensity exercise, lasting around one to four minutes, followed by a short period of recovery.[121] A total HIIT workout, including a warmup and cooldown usually lasts around 20-25 minutes and can be completed from home, a park, or even a spare meeting room in the office. Many of my busy clients find that squeezing in a short HIIT session at a time that works for them is much more doable than trying to make a class at the gym or committing to a long walk or run. It can be a great way to give you a quick burst of energy to break up your day.

You can follow a guided workout video or create a simple series of exercises using your own bodyweight. It doesn't have to be complicated or fancy. For example, you could complete one minute each of squats, pushups on your knees, jogging on the spot, and a plank hold with a 30-second rest in between each exercise, and repeated twice. With a minute of warming up and cooling down on either side, this whole sequence would take just 14 minutes but would increase your heart rate, boost your metabolism, and get lots of different muscle groups firing.

Contrary to popular belief, short HIIT-style workouts have been shown to be as effective at improving cardiovascular health and aerobic capacity as endurance-based cardio exercise (such as jogging or cycling).[119] This style of movement also has the added benefit of increasing your muscle's sensitivity to insulin, so is arguably more beneficial for women with PCOS.

That said, if you know that you don't enjoy HIIT workouts and love a longer jog, swim, or bike ride, then stick with it! The best form of exercise for your PCOS is the one that you will stick with in the long run.

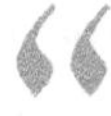

> So long as you feel energized afterward and aren't noticing negative impacts on your sleep, keep up any form of movement that makes you feel good.

Bonus points if you can tie your exercise to something you look forward to such as a catchup walk with a friend or dancing to your favorite music.

Incidental movement for the win

Some of the best forms of exercise to lower cortisol and inflammation and improve insulin resistance are low-intensity exercises like walking, gentle swimming, gardening, and playing with your kids. Aim to include as much of this in your day as possible. If you work at a desk, consider trialing a standing desk. Organize walking meetings or catch ups with friends. Park further away. Or take a walk around the block on your lunch break.

Let go of exercising to lose weight

For most of my life, I equated exercise with losing or maintaining my weight. If your PCOS diagnosis was anything like the majority of Cysters I've met, you were probably told to "eat less and exercise more." You likely found that exercise wasn't working, so you worked out harder and for longer, still with no results. It's no wonder working out has a negative connotation for so many Cysters.

It's time to let the calories in, calories out equation go. This *doesn't* apply for PCOS. When your root cause is ruling your body, it is almost impossible to lose weight, even when you are in a calorie deficit. By working on lowering your insulin, cortisol, and inflammation, you'll be able to move your body out of a place of danger and into one of safety. Once your body systems are working in harmony again, you will find weight loss is far more achievable. For a deep dive into weight loss in PCOS, I've put together a bonus resource for you: Simple Weight Loss Strategies for PCOS. Access your bonus resources at nourishednaturalhealth.com/resources

Can't start exercising? Try these three tricks

Sometimes getting into a routine with regular exercise can be really hard, even when you know it is helpful for your PCOS. Try these three simple tricks that have helped many of my clients:

Pack your bag the night before

It sounds trivial, but getting organized before going to bed at night can really help with motivation the next morning. If you are going to a gym class, pack your bag so you can grab it and go before letting the excuses creep in. If you exercise at home, lay your shoes and socks out next to your mat, fill a water bottle and decide on the routine you'll follow so you can simply hit play and get started.

The five-minute rule

The five-minute rule is a technique used in cognitive behavioral therapy to help with procrastination. You can use this in any area of your life where you struggle to get started, but it works particularly well with exercise. If you just can't start your workout because the idea of a full 20 minutes seems overwhelming, tell yourself you only have to commit to five.

Do just the first five minutes of a workout and then stop and assess. Do you think you could do another five? 99% of the time, you'll find that once you get going and the endorphins start flowing, you'll be able to keep going. If after the first five minutes you genuinely feel too tired to keep going – honor that. Your body knows what's best.

Exercise snacking

This technique works well if you genuinely don't have time to exercise because of your schedule. Instead of a formal exercise practice, try adding "snack sized" bursts of exercise throughout your day. For example, while you are waiting for the kettle to boil, do ten squats. While in the lift, do five calf raises (rise up from flat feet onto your toes and back down again). When you're on the phone, march on the spot or walk around the meeting room.

ACTION STEP:

What's your favorite PCOS-friendly type of exercise? Share with our community in the PCOS Repair Protocol Cysterhood community and check out what movement other Cysters are trying. Haven't created a free account yet? Go to nourishednaturalhealth.com/resources

Chapter 21

Getting Pregnant with PCOS

Many of you reading this book will be here because of your dream to fall pregnant with PCOS. Maybe you were told that you would struggle to fall pregnant naturally one day, or perhaps struggles with fertility caused your PCOS to be first diagnosed. Either way, I know firsthand how strong the desire to have a baby can be and how frustrating and disheartening it can feel to know that your PCOS could be slowing things down.

Firstly, I want you to know that despite what you might have been told, PCOS is *not* an infertility diagnosis. It is a condition of *subfertility* – meaning that it might take you longer to fall pregnant than another woman without PCOS, but it is absolutely possible.

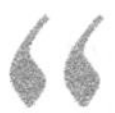

In fact, research shows that women with PCOS have, on average, the same number of children as women without PCOS.[122]

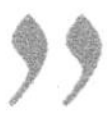

What's more, the majority of Cysters will have at least one natural pregnancy without needing any fertility treatments.[123] Research suggests that women with PCOS remain fertile for longer due to a higher ovarian reserve, meaning that you likely have longer to have children than your non-PCOS friends.[123]

I like to think about getting pregnant with PCOS as three steps:

1. Work out your PCOS root cause that is impacting your hormones, ovulation, and cycle length.
2. Reverse your root cause so that you can start ovulating naturally again.
3. Learn how to chart your cycles and time sex for conception.

By now, you are already doing step one and two. Remember, it usually takes several months for the powerful habit changes you are making to start to show in your cycle and other symptoms – so hang in there.

As a trained Fertility Educator, I have observed again and again how the simple skill of being able to identify ovulation is often the final missing link in falling pregnant naturally with PCOS. Women with PCOS rarely ovulate at the predicted time because our hormones cause our cycles to be a little wonky. This *doesn't* mean it's impossible to get pregnant, it just means we need to pay closer attention to signs like our cervical fluid to know when our body is gearing up to release an egg.

Learning to chart your cycles for fertility is a topic far beyond the scope of this book, but because I know how important it is for many of you, I didn't want to leave you hanging. I have created an in-depth mini course all about fertility and PCOS that I am including as a free bonus for you. In the four-part video series, I've outlined how to track your cycle (even if it's wonky or irregular), how to confirm you are ovulating, and how to time intercourse for pregnancy. You can access the PCOS Fertility Formula mini course via nourishednaturalhealth.com/resources

STEP FOUR: Find a Community

Beyond all of the food, mindset, supplement, and lifestyle changes we have covered so far, the PCOS Repair Protocol wouldn't be complete without talking about the importance of community. At the time of writing, a few years of lockdowns and isolations due to the COVID-19 pandemic has pushed many of us to our limit. Throughout all of our lives, due to various circumstances, there will be times when we struggle to find community, especially when we need it most. Personally, I found becoming a new mom in 2021 amidst a global pandemic to be one of the most isolating and lonely experiences in my life so far.

All humans are hardwired to seek connection with others, and this connection significantly impacts our health. Research shows that social support and feeling connected to others helps us to maintain a healthy weight, control blood sugar, decrease cardiovascular risks, and improve mental health.[124] Conversely, social isolation can increase depressive symptoms, decrease your lifespan, and quality of life.[124] In the words of psychiatrist Dr Hallowell, "just as we need vitamin C each day, we also need a dose of the human moment – positive contact with other people."[125]

It's connections with others and feeling part of something larger than ourselves that gets us through the tough times and gives meaning to the good. In a world focussed on achievement, productivity, and busyness, making time to connect with others can feel insignificant. However, strong connections make life more meaningful and improve your health.

There is something particularly gratifying about being part of a community of women. In many cultures, women traditionally spent large amounts of time together in groups menstruating, giving birth, looking after children, and finding support and encouragement from their mothers, sisters, and aunts.

Being diagnosed with PCOS can feel deeply isolating. Many of my clients who have struggled with fertility have shared with me that their diagnosis made them feel like less of a woman. That their body couldn't do what it was supposed to be born for. That they were broken. Every new pregnancy announcement on Facebook felt like a sharp stab in the back, reminding them of what they didn't have.

Each time my acne flared up, I wanted to crawl into a dark room and cancel every social plan I had for weeks. It felt like everyone around me had flawless skin and I couldn't bear the thought of them staring at my spots. I felt trapped in a body that was betraying me.

I know how alone you might feel in this syndrome, but I want you to know that there is an *incredible* community of women out there who are experiencing the same struggles as you are. Research shows that *at least* one in ten women of reproductive age have been diagnosed with PCOS, and many more remain undiagnosed. I urge you to seek out these women and connect with them on your healing journey.

I created a free support group for all readers of the PCOS Repair Protocol so that you can instantly access the support of other Cysters. If you haven't already, join the group at nourishednaturalhealth.com/resources. This group is a safe space for you to share your story, ask for help, laugh, cry, and learn from other Cysters. Most of all, it's a space to know that you aren't alone.

The bonds I have created with other women throughout my own journey have been integral to my healing. As the world closed down during the pandemic and in-person conversations became a distant memory, I realized the phenomenal importance of staying connected to others through digital platforms. Some of my strongest friendships are with women I have met online. What brought us together wasn't our geography but our shared experiences. There is nothing quite as powerful as being able to say "I get it. I've been there too."

SPOTLIGHT: Eunice's story - shared experience for healing

Eunice was one of the first members to complete my group program back in 2020 after living with PCOS for 10 years. After spending a decade feeling alone in her symptoms, being part of our supportive community was integral in her healing process. In a video she recorded after completing the program she shared:

"It's been fantastic having a large community of women who are experiencing similar symptoms and being able to talk about these things in a safe space inside our group... The catch ups that we've been having every Monday have been super helpful as well because we are able to ask questions directly to Tam. We get her opinion right there and then...and also get to hear the success stories from all the other lovely ladies who are joining - it has been incredible".

Watch Eunice's full story via nourishednaturalhealth.com/resources

Finding connections with others to support you on your journey doesn't have to be in online groups if that isn't your vibe. It could be a local in-person group. It could even be just one other friend who has PCOS or a similar health struggle who you stay in touch with. Whatever it is, if you can find a way of walking this path with others it will be infinitely easier and more enjoyable.

At this point, you have all the tools you need to heal the root cause of your PCOS. You know how to lower your androgens, identify your root cause, create an individualized protocol, and connect to a support community. For many women, this is enough. However, for those of you who, after reading this book, find you need help implementing the protocols, staying motivated, or digging deeper into your root cause, I created a completely customizable video course called the PCOS Repair Digital Program. Joining the 8-week program is the ultimate way to put your PCOS healing journey front and center and fast track your results.

Inside the program, we help you confirm your root cause (or combination of root causes in some situations). We do this through comprehensive quizzes as well as access to blood testing where necessary and assistance in interpreting your results. We then provide you with an individualized protocol so that you can focus only on the most impactful changes for your body. Members receive tons of support resources including recipes, workout videos, symptom troubleshooting, medication pros and cons and more.

To find out more, visit nourishednaturalhealth.com/resources

Chapter 22

Where To From Here? How To Keep Moving Forward

You now have all the tools you need to heal your root cause and start thriving with PCOS.

It's important to remember that we are striving for *progress* not perfection.

It's the habits and practices that you are consistent with over the years, not weeks, that determine your health. One day of eating poorly or a week of not following your morning routine isn't going to derail your progress. What's important is how quickly you are able to pick yourself up and come back to the principles that you know support your body and improve your life.

Now that you have the protocols to thrive with PCOS, the next step is to find ways to make these changes sustainable and enjoyable habits that you can stick with in the long run. It's important to balance the practices that serve our physical body (like eating lots of vegetables or doing regular exercise) with those that nourish our soul. Over the years, I have witnessed so many Cysters beat themselves up about eating a single ice cream or burger. The reality is the damage we can do through our negative self-talk can create far worse health outcomes than just eating the less nourishing food and getting on with it.

One of my favorite ways to create sustainable habits is to use the 80/20 rule. Following all of the recommendations in this book 100% of the time isn't realistic. If you have ever tried yo-yo dieting for your PCOS, you'll know this scenario all too well. Monday morning rolls around, you feel inspired and ready to stick to your new diet and exercise routine. It's going well all week, and then Friday rolls around. You are missing your favorite foods, and you're hungry, tired, and cranky. Someone at work brings chocolate and you think "I'll just have one – I've been so good all week." Then, before you know it, you've polished off a bag of chips on your way home, decided "It's all ruined now anyway," and ordered pizza for dinner.

Instead of this *all or nothing* approach, I want you to focus on following the PCOS Repair Protocol principles for your root cause 80% of the time. Then, for the other 20%, choose foods and practices that fill your soul. I like to call these "soul foods."

For example, if you have Insulin-Resistant PCOS, you might eat the high protein breakfast from Monday to Saturday, and then on Sunday, treat yourself to brunch with friends where you can order anything you feel like on the menu. If you have Inflammatory PCOS and are trialing removing gluten and dairy from your diet, you might eat strictly gluten and dairy free during the week and then indulge in a delicious pastry or fresh baguette on the weekend. You might be following the

HIIT workout principles most days, but one morning wake up craving connection so decide to give yourself a morning off and go for a coffee with a friend instead.

Following the 80/20 rule means you never feel deprived because you know that just around the corner is an opportunity to choose what you are truly craving, even if it might not be the best for your PCOS. This means that when you do indulge in "soul food," you are much less likely to overeat or spiral out of control.

Feeling restricted means that when we do finally give in to our cravings, we often have the mentality of "screw it – I've already ruined it, I might as well keep going." Make a mental list of your favorite things to eat and do. Instead of trying to avoid these entirely, I want you to *plan* for when you will include these in your week. Make it a big deal and really be present while you enjoy them.

How long do I need to keep taking the supplements?

I suggest remaining on your Root Cause Core Treatment supplements for around three to four months. At this point, it is a good idea to visit your doctor to have some testing done to assess your root cause. For example, you might check your insulin levels, inflammatory markers, thyroid panel, or cortisol. If your test results show that your root cause has been reversed (for example, you are no longer insulin-resistant), or your symptoms have greatly improved, you can drop down to a maintenance dose.

This might look like taking your current supplements once every second day or dropping the daily dose to 50%. After another four weeks, reassess how you are feeling. You will likely be able to stop most of your supplements and maintain your results through diet, movement, and the other lifestyle changes we have covered in this book.

Once your symptoms have resolved significantly and you are no longer noticing hangry attacks, sugar cravings, and energy crashes throughout the day, you can experiment with reducing the protein in your breakfast as well. You might find that you don't need to follow the Repair Breakfast principles as closely because your insulin is now much more balanced.

If you still have symptoms or your test results show your root cause hasn't been reversed after three to four months, I suggest continuing with your current supplement regime and Root Cause Core Treatment. You might like to take a short break from your supplements for one to two weeks every few months to give your body a break.

We're in this for the long haul

For most Cysters, PCOS takes time to heal. Depending on how significant your root cause was when you started implementing the PCOS Repair Protocol, it's not uncommon for it to take around six months before you see considerable changes to your symptoms.

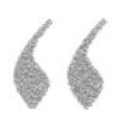

> Remember – small changes add up to big impact over time.

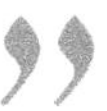

The changes we've made together over the last few weeks aren't a quick fix. They won't resolve your symptoms overnight. This approach requires consistent effort, but the changes you see will be powerful and long lasting.

If you feel called to dig deeper and continue learning how to support your unique root cause, join us in the PCOS Repair Digital Program. Our community is bursting with other Cysters like you who are saying "YES!" to putting their health first and thriving with PCOS, not despite it. Find out more at nourishednaturalhealth.com/resources

Final Thoughts

I hope that this book has helped you see that PCOS is not a life sentence of suffering. You are not a victim to a body that is betraying you. You are no less of a woman. You certainly aren't broken.

You have an incredible gift – the ultimate wake-up call to take charge of your life. To fill your own cup so that you can be the brightest version of yourself and positively impact those around you.

Your body is incredibly intelligent at communicating its needs to you through symptoms. This journey has already made you healthier, stronger, more compassionate, and resilient.

You *can* live a life of abundance and potential. You already have all the tools you need inside you to shift your reality from suffering to thriving.

You have the strength of one of the most supportive communities of women behind you.

It's time to lean in and take control again, Cyster.

Resources and Links

All resources and links mentioned in this book can be access via nourishednaturalhealth.com/resources

There you will find more than $900 worth of free bonuses, the link to join our free support community, information about the 8-week digital program and all vitamins mentioned for specific root causes throughout the book.

If you need help accessing these resources at any time, please feel free to reach out to our friendly support team at hello@ nourishednaturalhealth.com

I can't wait to continue to support you on your journey.

I need your help

If you found this book helpful it would mean so much to me if you leave a review on Amazon or Goodreads.

It is my life calling to get this information into the hands of as many women as physically (or digitally!) possible. I believe that all women deserve access to this life changing information.

By leaving a review you will help the women who need this book see that it can change their lives for the better. No matter what, I appreciate you and can't wait to continue to support you on your journey.

As you continue to implement the Protocol, don't forget to share your journey in our PCOS Repair Cysterhood Community or tag me on Instagram @nourishednaturalhealth so that we can all cheer you on.

Here's to you, Cyster.

References

1. Teede HJ, Norman RJ, Garad RM. A new evidence-based guideline for assessment and management of polycystic ovary syndrome. *Med J Aust.* 2019;210(6):285-285.e1.

2. Kristensen SL, Ramlau-Hansen CH, Ernst E, et al. A very large proportion of young Danish women have polycystic ovaries: is a revision of the Rotterdam criteria needed? *Hum Reprod.* 2010;25(12):3117-3122.

3. Azziz R. Polycystic ovary syndrome: what's in a name? *J Clin Endocrinol Metab.* 2014;99(4):1142-1145.

4. Yilmaz B, Vellanki P, Ata B, Yildiz BO. Metabolic syndrome, hypertension, and hyperlipidemia in mothers, fathers, sisters, and brothers of women with polycystic ovary syndrome: a systematic review and meta-analysis. *Fertil Steril.* 2018;109(2):356-364.e32.

5. Palioura E, Diamanti-Kandarakis E. Polycystic ovary syndrome (PCOS) and endocrine disrupting chemicals (EDCs). *Rev Endocr Metab Disord.* 2015;16(4):365-371.

6. Steegers-Theunissen RPM, Wiegel RE, Jansen PW, Laven JSE, Sinclair KD. Polycystic Ovary Syndrome: A Brain Disorder Characterized by Eating Problems Originating during Puberty and Adolescence. *Int J Mol Sci.* 2020;21(21):8211.

7. Dapas M, Lin FTJ, Nadkarni GN, et al. Distinct subtypes of polycystic ovary syndrome with novel genetic associations: An unsupervised, phenotypic clustering analysis. *PLoS Med.* 2020;17(6):e1003132.

8. Niethammer B, Körner C, Schmidmayr M, Luppa PB, Seifert-Klauss VR. Non-reproductive Effects of Anovulation: Bone Metabolism in the Luteal

Phase of Premenopausal Women Differs between Ovulatory and Anovulatory Cycles. *Geburtshilfe Frauenheilkd*. 2015;75(12):1250-1257.

9. Mastrogiannis DS, Spiliopoulos M, Mulla W, Homko CJ. Insulin resistance: The possible link between gestational diabetes mellitus and hypertensive disorders of pregnancy. *Curr Diab Rep*. 2009;9(4):296.

10. Fica S, Albu A, Constantin M, Dobri GA. Insulin resistance and fertility in polycystic ovary syndrome. *J Med Life*. 2008///Oct-Dec;1(4):415-422.

11. Furman D, Campisi J, Verdin E, et al. Chronic inflammation in the etiology of disease across the life span. *Nat Med*. 2019;25(12):1822-1832.

12. Wu C, Wei K, Jiang Z. 5α-reductase activity in women with polycystic ovary syndrome: a systematic review and meta-analysis. *Reprod Biol Endocrinol*. 2017;15(1):21-21.

13. Mehraban M, Jelodar G, Rahmanifar F. A combination of spearmint and flaxseed extract improved endocrine and histomorphology of ovary in experimental PCOS. *J Ovarian Res*. 2020;13(1):32.

14. Grant P. Spearmint herbal tea has significant anti-androgen effects in polycystic ovarian syndrome. A randomized controlled trial. *Phytother Res*. 2010;24(2):186-188.

15. Bandariyan E, Mogheiseh A, Ahmadi A. The effect of lutein and Urtica dioica extract on in vitro production of embryo and oxidative status in polycystic ovary syndrome in a model of mice. *BMC Complementary Medicine and Therapies*. 2021;21(1):55.

16. Chen JT, Tominaga K, Sato Y, Anzai H, Matsuoka R. Maitake mushroom (Grifola frondosa) extract induces ovulation in patients with polycystic ovary syndrome: a possible monotherapy and a combination therapy after failure with first-line clomiphene citrate. *J Altern Complement Med*. 2010;16(12):1295-1299.

17. Grant P, Ramasamy S. An update on plant derived anti-androgens. *Int J Endocrinol Metab*. 2012;10(2):497-502.

18. Fujita R, Liu J, Shimizu K, et al. Anti-androgenic activities of Ganoderma lucidum. *J Ethnopharmacol*. 2005;102(1):107-112.

19. Stamatiadis D, Bulteau-Portois MC, Mowszowicz I. Inhibition of 5 alpha-reductase activity in human skin by zinc and azelaic acid. *Br J Dermatol.* 1988;119(5):627-632.

20. Unfer V, Nestler JE, Kamenov ZA, Prapas N, Facchinetti F. Effects of Inositol(s) in Women with PCOS: A Systematic Review of Randomized Controlled Trials. *Int J Endocrinol.* 2016;2016:1849162-1849162.

21. Abdel Hamid AMS, Ismail Madkour WA, Borg TF. Inositol versus Metformin administration in polycystic ovary syndrome patients: a case–control study. *Journal of Evidence-Based Women's Health Journal Society.* 2015;5(3). https://journals.lww.com/ebjwh/Fulltext/2015/08000/Inositol_versus_Metformin_administration_in.2.aspx

22. Jakubowicz D, Barnea M, Wainstein J, Froy O. Effects of caloric intake timing on insulin resistance and hyperandrogenism in lean women with polycystic ovary syndrome. *Clin Sci.* 2013;125(9):423-432.

23. Zhang W, Wang X, Liu Y, et al. Effects of dietary flaxseed lignan extract on symptoms of benign prostatic hyperplasia. *J Med Food.* 2008;11(2):207-214.

24. Nowak DA, Snyder DC, Brown AJ, Demark-Wahnefried W. The Effect of Flaxseed Supplementation on Hormonal Levels Associated with Polycystic Ovarian Syndrome: A Case Study. *Curr Top Nutraceutical Res.* 2007;5(4):177-181.

25. Ulrich J, Goerges J, Keck C, Müller-Wieland D, Diederich S, Janssen OE. Impact of Autoimmune Thyroiditis on Reproductive and Metabolic Parameters in Patients with Polycystic Ovary Syndrome. *Exp Clin Endocrinol Diabetes.* 2018;126(4):198-204.

26. Singla R, Gupta Y, Khemani M, Aggarwal S. Thyroid disorders and polycystic ovary syndrome: An emerging relationship. *Indian J Endocrinol Metab.* 2015/// Jan-Feb;19(1):25-29.

27. Hadi A, Pourmasoumi M, Najafgholizadeh A, Clark CCT, Esmaillzadeh A. The effect of apple cider vinegar on lipid profiles and glycemic parameters: a systematic review and meta-analysis of randomized clinical trials. *BMC complementary medicine and therapies.* 2021;21(1):179-179.

28. Urtasun R, Díaz-Gómez J, Araña M, et al. A Combination of Apple Vinegar Drink with Bacillus coagulans Ameliorates High Fat Diet-Induced Body Weight Gain, Insulin Resistance and Hepatic Steatosis. *Nutrients*. 2020;12(9):2504.

29. Maleki V, Taheri E, Varshosaz P, et al. A comprehensive insight into effects of green tea extract in polycystic ovary syndrome: a systematic review. *Reprod Biol Endocrinol*. 2021;19(1):147.

30. Tehrani HG, Allahdadian M, Zarre F, Ranjbar H, Allahdadian F. Effect of green tea on metabolic and hormonal aspect of polycystic ovarian syndrome in overweight and obese women suffering from polycystic ovarian syndrome: A clinical trial. *J Educ Health Promot*. 2017;6:36-36.

31. Wang JG, Anderson RA, Graham GM 3rd, et al. The effect of cinnamon extract on insulin resistance parameters in polycystic ovary syndrome: a pilot study. *Fertil Steril*. 2007;88(1):240-243.

32. Heshmati J, Sepidarkish M, Morvaridzadeh M, et al. The effect of cinnamon supplementation on glycemic control in women with polycystic ovary syndrome: A systematic review and meta-analysis. *J Food Biochem*. 2020;45(1):e13543.

33. Chien YJ, Chang CY, Wu MY, Chen CH, Horng YS, Wu HC. Effects of Curcumin on Glycemic Control and Lipid Profile in Polycystic Ovary Syndrome: Systematic Review with Meta-Analysis and Trial Sequential Analysis. *Nutrients*. 2021;13(2):684.

34. Zhao X, Jiang Y, Xi H, Chen L, Feng X. Exploration of the Relationship Between Gut Microbiota and Polycystic Ovary Syndrome (PCOS): a Review. *Geburtshilfe Frauenheilkd*. 2020;80(2):161-171.

35. Thota RN, Acharya SH, Garg ML. Curcumin and/or omega-3 polyunsaturated fatty acids supplementation reduces insulin resistance and blood lipids in individuals with high risk of type 2 diabetes: a randomised controlled trial. *Lipids Health Dis*. 2019;18(1):31.

36. Jung JY, Kwon HH, Hong JS, et al. Effect of dietary supplementation with omega-3 fatty acid and gamma-linolenic acid on acne vulgaris: a randomised, double-blind, controlled trial. *Acta Derm Venereol*. 2014;94(5):521-525.

37. Zuo T, Zhu M, Xu W. Roles of Oxidative Stress in Polycystic Ovary Syndrome and Cancers. *Oxid Med Cell Longev*. 2015;2016:8589318.

38. Briden L. *The Period Repair Manual.* CreateSpace Independent Publishing Platform; 2017.

39. DeUgarte CM, Bartolucci AA, Azziz R. Prevalence of insulin resistance in the polycystic ovary syndrome using the homeostasis model assessment. *Fertil Steril.* 2005;83(5):1454-1460.

40. Stepto NK, Cassar S, Joham AE, et al. Women with polycystic ovary syndrome have intrinsic insulin resistance on euglycaemic-hyperinsulaemic clamp. *Hum Reprod.* 2013;28(3):777-784.

41. Dunaif A. Insulin resistance and the polycystic ovary syndrome: mechanism and implications for pathogenesis. *Endocr Rev.* 1997;18(6):774-800.

42. Franks S, Stark J, Hardy K. Follicle dynamics and anovulation in polycystic ovary syndrome. *Hum Reprod Update.* 2008;14(4):367-378.

43. Guo F, Moellering DR, Garvey WT. Use of HbA1c for diagnoses of diabetes and prediabetes: comparison with diagnoses based on fasting and 2-hr glucose values and effects of gender, race, and age. *Metab Syndr Relat Disord.* 2014;12(5):258-268.

44. Tirosh A, Shai I, Tekes-Manova D, et al. Normal Fasting Plasma Glucose Levels and Type 2 Diabetes in Young Men. *N Engl J Med.* 2005;353(14):1454-1462.

45. Kraft JR. Detection of Diabetes Mellitus In Situ (Occult Diabetes). *Lab Med.* 1975;6(2):10-22.

46. DiNicolantonio JJ, Bhutani J, OKeefe JH, Crofts C. Postprandial insulin assay as the earliest biomarker for diagnosing pre-diabetes, type 2 diabetes and increased cardiovascular risk. *Open Heart.* 2017;4(2):e000656.

47. Siavash M, Tabbakhian M, Sabzghabaee AM, Razavi N. Severity of Gastrointestinal Side Effects of Metformin Tablet Compared to Metformin Capsule in Type 2 Diabetes Mellitus Patients. *Journal of research in pharmacy practice.* 2017///Apr-Jun;6(2):73-76.

48. Softic S, Stanhope KL, Boucher J, et al. Fructose and hepatic insulin resistance. *Crit Rev Clin Lab Sci.* 2020;57(5):308-322.

49. Donga E, van Dijk M, van Dijk JG, et al. A single night of partial sleep deprivation induces insulin resistance in multiple metabolic pathways in healthy subjects. *J Clin Endocrinol Metab.* 2010;95(6):2963-2968.

50. Venkatasamy VV, Pericherla S, Manthuruthil S, Mishra S, Hanno R. Effect of Physical activity on Insulin Resistance, Inflammation and Oxidative Stress in Diabetes Mellitus. *J Clin Diagn Res.* 2013;7(8):1764-1766.

51. Entringer S, Wüst S, Kumsta R, et al. Prenatal psychosocial stress exposure is associated with insulin resistance in young adults. *Am J Obstet Gynecol.* 2008;199(5):498.e1-e7.

52. Garcia-Vargas L, Addison SS, Nistala R, Kurukulasuriya D, Sowers JR. Gestational Diabetes and the Offspring: Implications in the Development of the Cardiorenal Metabolic Syndrome in Offspring. *Cardiorenal Med.* 2012;2(2):134-142.

53. Caricilli AM, Saad MJA. The role of gut microbiota on insulin resistance. *Nutrients.* 2013;5(3):829-851.

54. Yildiz BO, Azziz R. The adrenal and polycystic ovary syndrome. *Rev Endocr Metab Disord.* 2007;8(4):331-342.

55. Christodoulaki C, Trakakis E, Pergialiotis V, et al. Dehydroepiandrosterone-Sulfate, Insulin Resistance and Ovarian Volume Estimation in Patients With Polycystic Ovarian Syndrome. *J Family Reprod Health.* 2017;11(1):24-29.

56. Deng Y, Zhang Y, Li S, et al. Steroid hormone profiling in obese and nonobese women with polycystic ovary syndrome. *Sci Rep.* 2017;7(1):14156-14156.

57. Stewart ME, Greenwood R, Cunliffe WJ, Strauss JS, Downing DT. Effect of cyproterone acetate-ethinyl estradiol treatment on the proportions of linoleic and sebaleic acids in various skin surface lipid classes. *Arch Dermatol Res.* 1986;278(6):481-485.

58. Cortés ME, Alfaro AA. The effects of hormonal contraceptives on glycemic regulation. *Linacre Q.* 2014;81(3):209-218.

59. Khalili H. Risk of Inflammatory Bowel Disease with Oral Contraceptives and Menopausal Hormone Therapy: Current Evidence and Future Directions. *Drug Saf.* 2016;39(3):193-197.

60. Jobira B, Frank DN, Pyle L, et al. Obese Adolescents With PCOS Have Altered Biodiversity and Relative Abundance in Gastrointestinal Microbiota. *J Clin Endocrinol Metab.* 2020;105(6):e2134-e2144.

61. Rudnicka E, Suchta K, Grymowicz M, et al. Chronic Low Grade Inflammation in Pathogenesis of PCOS. *Int J Mol Sci*. 2021;22(7). doi:10.3390/ijms22073789

62. González F. Inflammation in Polycystic Ovary Syndrome: underpinning of insulin resistance and ovarian dysfunction. *Steroids*. 2012;77(4):300-305.

63. Garelli S, Masiero S, Plebani M, et al. High prevalence of chronic thyroiditis in patients with polycystic ovary syndrome. *Eur J Obstet Gynecol Reprod Biol*. 2013;169(2):248-251.

64. Harvey LJ, Armah CN, Dainty JR, et al. Impact of menstrual blood loss and diet on iron deficiency among women in the UK. *Br J Nutr*. 2005;94(4):557-564.

65. Wessling-Resnick M. Iron homeostasis and the inflammatory response. *Annu Rev Nutr*. 2010;30:105-122.

66. Rotterdam ESHRE/ASRM-Sponsored PCOS Consensus Workshop Group. Revised 2003 consensus on diagnostic criteria and long-term health risks related to polycystic ovary syndrome. *Fertil Steril*. 2004;81(1):19-25.

67. Rachoń D. Differential diagnosis of hyperandrogenism in women with polycystic ovary syndrome. *Exp Clin Endocrinol Diabetes*. 2012;120(4):205-209.

68. Ashraf S, Nabi M, Rasool S ul A, Rashid F, Amin S. Hyperandrogenism in polycystic ovarian syndrome and role of CYP gene variants: a review. *Egyptian Journal of Medical Human Genetics*. 2019;20(1):25.

69. McGrice M, Porter J. The Effect of Low Carbohydrate Diets on Fertility Hormones and Outcomes in Overweight and Obese Women: A Systematic Review. *Nutrients*. 2017;9(3):204.

70. Mady MA, Kossoff EH, McGregor AL, Wheless JW, Pyzik PL, Freeman JM. The ketogenic diet: adolescents can do it, too. *Epilepsia*. 2003;44(6):847-851.

71. Tappy L, Rosset R. Health outcomes of a high fructose intake: the importance of physical activity. *J Physiol*. 2019;597(14):3561-3571.

72. Jang C, Hui S, Lu W, et al. The Small Intestine Converts Dietary Fructose into Glucose and Organic Acids. *Cell Metab*. 2018;27(2):351-361.e3.

73. Shi YN, Liu YJ, Xie Z, Zhang WJ. Fructose and metabolic diseases: too much to be good. *Chin Med J*. 2021;134(11):1276-1285.

74. Chiofalo B, Laganà AS, Palmara V, et al. Fasting as possible complementary approach for polycystic ovary syndrome: Hope or hype? *Med Hypotheses.* 2017;105:1-3.

75. Moini Jazani A, Nasimi Doost Azgomi H, Nasimi Doost Azgomi A, Nasimi Doost Azgomi R. A comprehensive review of clinical studies with herbal medicine on polycystic ovary syndrome (PCOS). *Daru.* 2019;27(2):863-877.

76. Morais JBS, Severo JS, de Alencar GRR, et al. Effect of magnesium supplementation on insulin resistance in humans: A systematic review. *Nutrition.* 2017;38:54-60.

77. Anton SD, Morrison CD, Cefalu WT, et al. Effects of chromium picolinate on food intake and satiety. *Diabetes Technol Ther.* 2008;10(5):405-412.

78. Tandon N, Yadav SS. Safety and clinical effectiveness of Withania Somnifera (Linn.) Dunal root in human ailments. *J Ethnopharmacol.* 2020;255:112768.

79. Durg S, Bavage S, Shivaram SB. Withania somnifera (Indian ginseng) in diabetes mellitus: A systematic review and meta-analysis of scientific evidence from experimental research to clinical application. *Phytother Res.* 2020;34(5):1041-1059.

80. Markus R, Panhuysen G, Tuiten A, Koppeschaar H. Effects of food on cortisol and mood in vulnerable subjects under controllable and uncontrollable stress. *Physiol Behav.* 2000;70(3-4):333-342.

81. Bravo JA, Forsythe P, Chew MV, et al. Ingestion of Lactobacillus strain regulates emotional behavior and central GABA receptor expression in a mouse via the vagus nerve. *Proc Natl Acad Sci U S A.* 2011;108(38):16050-16055.

82. Ulvestad M, Bjertness E, Dalgard F, Halvorsen JA. Acne and dairy products in adolescence: results from a Norwegian longitudinal study. *J Eur Acad Dermatol Venereol.* 2016;31(3):530-535.

83. Melnik BC. Diet in acne: further evidence for the role of nutrient signalling in acne pathogenesis. *Acta Derm Venereol.* 2012;92(3):228-231.

84. Palmery M, Saraceno A, Vaiarelli A, Carlomagno G. Oral contraceptives and changes in nutritional requirements. *Eur Rev Med Pharmacol Sci.* 2013;17(13):1804-1813.

85. Cervantes J, Eber AE, Perper M, Nascimento VM, Nouri K, Keri JE. The role of zinc in the treatment of acne: A review of the literature. *Dermatol Ther.* 2017;31(1). doi:10.1111/dth.12576

86. Bowe WP, Logan AC. Acne vulgaris, probiotics and the gut-brain-skin axis – back to the future? *Gut Pathog.* 2011;3(1):1-1.

87. Takeyama M, Nagareda T, Takatsuka D, et al. Stimulatory effect of prolactin on luteinizing hormone-induced testicular 5 alpha-reductase activity in hypophysectomized adult rats. *Endocrinology.* 1986;118(6):2268-2275.

88. Sinha U, Sinharay K, Saha S, Longkumer TA, Baul SN, Pal SK. Thyroid disorders in polycystic ovarian syndrome subjects: A tertiary hospital based cross-sectional study from Eastern India. *Indian J Endocrinol Metab.* 2013;17(2):304-309.

89. Deyneli O, Akpınar IN, Meriçliler OS, Gözü H, Yıldız ME, Akalın NS. Effects of levothyroxine treatment on insulin sensitivity, endothelial function and risk factors of atherosclerosis in hypothyroid women. *Ann Endocrinol.* 2014;75(4):220-226.

90. Kust D, Matesa N. The impact of familial predisposition on the development of Hashimoto's thyroiditis. *Acta Clin Belg.* 2018;75(2):104-108.

91. Orouji Jokar T, Fourman LT, Lee H, Mentzinger K, Fazeli PK. Higher TSH Levels Within the Normal Range Are Associated With Unexplained Infertility. *J Clin Endocrinol Metab.* 2018;103(2):632-639.

92. Kratzsch J, Fiedler GM, Leichtle A, et al. New reference intervals for thyrotropin and thyroid hormones based on National Academy of Clinical Biochemistry criteria and regular ultrasonography of the thyroid. *Clin Chem.* 2005;51(8):1480-1486.

93. Chen S, Zhou X, Zhu H, et al. Preconception TSH and pregnancy outcomes: a population-based cohort study in 184 611 women. *Clin Endocrinol.* 2017;86(6):816-824.

94. Liontiris MI, Mazokopakis EE. A concise review of Hashimoto thyroiditis (HT) and the importance of iodine, selenium, vitamin D and gluten on the autoimmunity and dietary management of HT patients.Points that need more investigation. *Hell J Nucl Med.* 2017;20(1):51-56.

95. Sategna-Guidetti C, Volta U, Ciacci C, et al. Prevalence of thyroid disorders in untreated adult celiac disease patients and effect of gluten withdrawal: an Italian multicenter study. *Am J Gastroenterol.* 2001;96(3):751-757.

96. Panda S, Kar A. Changes in thyroid hormone concentrations after administration of ashwagandha root extract to adult male mice. *J Pharm Pharmacol.* 1998;50(9):1065-1068.

97. Torres PJ, Siakowska M, Banaszewska B, et al. Gut Microbial Diversity in Women With Polycystic Ovary Syndrome Correlates With Hyperandrogenism. *J Clin Endocrinol Metab.* 2018;103(4):1502-1511.

98. Lam YY, Ha CWY, Campbell CR, et al. Increased gut permeability and microbiota change associate with mesenteric fat inflammation and metabolic dysfunction in diet-induced obese mice. *PLoS One.* 2012;7(3):e34233.

99. Farré R, Fiorani M, Abdu Rahiman S, Matteoli G. Intestinal Permeability, Inflammation and the Role of Nutrients. *Nutrients.* 2020;12(4):1185.

100. Lerner A, Ramesh A, Matthias T. Going gluten free in non-celiac autoimmune diseases: the missing ingredient. *Expert Rev Clin Immunol.* 2018;14(11):873-875.

101. Di Sabatino A, Volta U, Salvatore C, et al. Small Amounts of Gluten in Subjects With Suspected Nonceliac Gluten Sensitivity: A Randomized, Double-Blind, Placebo-Controlled, Cross-Over Trial. *Clin Gastroenterol Hepatol.* 2015;13(9):1604-1612.e3.

102. Mohammadi S, Kayedpoor P, Karimzadeh-Bardei L, Nabiuni M. The Effect of Curcumin on TNF-α, IL-6 and CRP Expression in a Model of Polycystic Ovary Syndrome as an Inflammation State. *Journal of reproduction & infertility.* 2017///Oct-Dec;18(4):352-360.

103. Ford ES, Cogswell ME. Diabetes and serum ferritin concentration among U.S. adults. *Diabetes Care.* 1999;22(12):1978-1983.

104. Thompson PA, Khatami M, Baglole CJ, et al. Environmental immune disruptors, inflammation and cancer risk. *Carcinogenesis.* 2015;36 Suppl 1(Suppl 1):S232-S253.

105. Dirty Dozen EWG's 2021 Shopper's Guide to Pesticides in Produce. Environmental Working Group. https://www.ewg.org/foodnews/dirty-dozen.php

106. Dantas WS, Neves W das, Gil S, et al. Exercise-induced anti-inflammatory effects in overweight/obese women with polycystic ovary syndrome. *Cytokine.* 2019;120:66-70.

107. Sapone A, Lammers KM, Mazzarella G, et al. Differential mucosal IL-17 expression in two gliadin-induced disorders: gluten sensitivity and the autoimmune enteropathy celiac disease. *Int Arch Allergy Immunol.* 2009;152(1):75-80.

108. Van Heertum K, Rossi B. Alcohol and fertility: how much is too much? *Fertility research and practice.* 2017;3:10-10.

109. Thomson RL, Spedding S, Buckley JD. Vitamin D in the aetiology and management of polycystic ovary syndrome. *Clin Endocrinol.* 2012;77(3):343-350.

110. Lin MW, Wu MH. The role of vitamin D in polycystic ovary syndrome. *Indian J Med Res.* 2015;142(3):238-240.

111. Alvarez JA, Ashraf A. Role of vitamin d in insulin secretion and insulin sensitivity for glucose homeostasis. *Int J Endocrinol.* 2010;2010:351385.

112. Butts SF, Seifer DB, Koelper N, et al. Vitamin D Deficiency Is Associated With Poor Ovarian Stimulation Outcome in PCOS but Not Unexplained Infertility. *J Clin Endocrinol Metab.* 2019;104(2):369-378.

113. Hamilton KP, Zelig R, Parker AR, Haggag A. Insulin Resistance and Serum Magnesium Concentrations among Women with Polycystic Ovary Syndrome. *Current developments in nutrition.* 2019;3(11):nzz108-nzz108.

114. DiNicolantonio JJ, O'Keefe JH, Wilson W. Subclinical magnesium deficiency: a principal driver of cardiovascular disease and a public health crisis. *Open heart.* 2018;5(1):e000668-e000668.

115. Lima M de L, Pousada J, Barbosa C, Cruz T. [Magnesium deficiency and insulin resistance in patients with type 2 diabetes mellitus]. *Arq Bras Endocrinol Metabol.* 2006;49(6):959-963.

116. Dzierzewski JM, Donovan EK, Kay DB, Sannes TS, Bradbrook KE. Sleep Inconsistency and Markers of Inflammation. *Front Neurol.* 2020;11. https://www.frontiersin.org/article/10.3389/fneur.2020.01042

117. Alizadeh M, Karandish M, Asghari Jafarabadi M, et al. Metabolic and hormonal effects of melatonin and/or magnesium supplementation in women with

polycystic ovary syndrome: a randomized, double-blind, placebo-controlled trial. *Nutr Metab.* 2021;18(1):57.

118. Mojaverrostami S, Asghari N, Khamisabadi M, Heidari Khoei H. The role of melatonin in polycystic ovary syndrome: A review. *International journal of reproductive biomedicine.* 2019;17(12):865-882.

119. Hill EE, Zack E, Battaglini C, Viru M, Viru A, Hackney AC. Exercise and circulating cortisol levels: the intensity threshold effect. *J Endocrinol Invest.* 2008;31(7):587-591.

120. Monash University. International evidence-based guideline for the assessment and management of polycystic ovary syndrome 2018. Jean Hailes. https://assets.jeanhailes.org.au/Tools/PCOS_evidence-based_guideline_for_assessment_and_management_pcos.pdf

121. Gaesser GA, Angadi SS. High-intensity interval training for health and fitness: can less be more? *J Appl Physiol.* 2011;111(6):1540-1541.

122. Joham AE, Boyle JA, Ranasinha S, Zoungas S, Teede HJ. Contraception use and pregnancy outcomes in women with polycystic ovary syndrome: data from the Australian Longitudinal Study on Women's Health. *Hum Reprod.* 2014;29(4):802-808.

123. Hudecova M, Holte J, Olovsson M, Sundström Poromaa I. Long-term follow-up of patients with polycystic ovary syndrome: reproductive outcome and ovarian reserve. *Hum Reprod.* 2009;24(5):1176-1183.

124. Martino J, Pegg J, Frates EP. The Connection Prescription: Using the Power of Social Interactions and the Deep Desire for Connectedness to Empower Health and Wellness. *Am J Lifestyle Med.* 2015;11(6):466-475.

125. Hallowell EM. *Connect: 12 Vital Ties That Open Your Heart, Lengthen Your Life, and Deepen Your Soul.* Simon and Schuster; 2001.